# Pleural Ultrasound for Clinicians

A TEXT AND E-BOOK

# Pleural Ultrasound for Clinicians

## A text and E-book

Edited by Claire L Tobin and Y C Gary Lee

Fergus Gleeson, David Feller-Kopman, and Najib Rahman

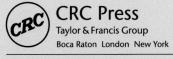

CRC Press
Taylor & Francis Group
Boca Raton  London  New York

CRC Press is an imprint of the
Taylor & Francis Group, an **informa** business

CRC Press
Taylor & Francis Group
6000 Broken Sound Parkway NW, Suite 300
Boca Raton, FL 33487-2742

First issued in paperback 2020

© 2014 by Taylor & Francis Group, LLC
CRC Press is an imprint of Taylor & Francis Group, an Informa business

No claim to original U.S. Government works

Version Date: 20130911

ISBN 13 : 978-0-367-57615-8 (pbk)
ISBN 13 : 978-1-4441-6695-8 (hbk)

**Library of Congress Cataloging-in-Publication Data**

Pleural ultrasound for clinicians : a text and e-book / editors, Y.C. Gary Lee, Claire Tobin, Fergus Gleeson,
   Najib Rahman, and David Feller-Kopman.
   p. ; cm.
   Includes bibliographical references.
   ISBN 978-1-4441-6695-8 (hardcover : alk. paper)
   I. Lee, Y. C. Gary, editor of compilation. II. Tobin, Claire, editor of compilation. III. Gleeson, Fergus, editor of
   compilation. IV. Rahman, Najib, editor of compilation. V. Feller-Kopman, David J., editor of compilation.
   [DNLM: 1. Pleural Diseases-- ultrasonography. 2. Ultrasonography-- methods. WF 141]

RC751
616.2'507543-- dc23                                                                          2013035481

Printed in the UK by Severn, Gloucester on responsibly sourced paper

**Visit the Taylor & Francis Web site at**
**http://www.taylorandfrancis.com**
**and the CRC Press Web site at**
**http://www.crcpress.com**

# Contents

# Preface

ULTRASOUND is an exciting imaging modality that allows portability, flexibility, and real-time dynamic imaging. Its use in thoracic medicine is expanding rapidly, particularly in the field of pleural disease. Use of pleural ultrasonography is increasingly recognized worldwide as an invaluable tool in the diagnosis and management of pleural patients at the bedside, significantly improving the efficiency and quality of patient care. Its use in guiding pleural intervention is now mandatory in many countries.

Proficiency in pleural ultrasound is a training requirement for respiratory specialists in a growing number of countries. Adequate training is the key to its successful application and use in clinical practice. This book is the first of its kind to fill the training needs for chest physicians and other non-radiologists, of all levels of experience, by providing essential knowledge on all aspects of pleural ultrasound in this new era. Understanding the basic principles of ultrasonography, its limitations, and commonly encountered artifacts is a crucial first step, as there is greater potential than with other forms of imaging for misinterpretation. Its skillful use can then be acquired at the bedside, with a designated mentor, through regular practice.

This book is written by chest physicians, with expert advice from internationally acclaimed thoracic radiologists. The authors are all enthusiastic teachers with many years of experience in running pleural ultrasound courses around the world. Their insight into the training needs of non-radiologists make this book unique.

This concise text is prepared with a clear clinical focus, to guide use of pleural ultrasound and enhance patient care. It delivers an extensive number of high-quality, original, real-time ultrasound images and teaching videos, carefully selected from the wide collections of the authors. We feel this provides the best learning media for readers to build an essential platform in acquiring the necessary skills in pleural ultrasound. Please refer to the E-book to view the ultrasound clips and teaching videos where you see a U or V symbol and where indicated in the caption. URLs also guide you to the ultrasound images and teaching videos should you prefer to access them this way. We feel this provides the best learning media for readers to build an essential platform in acquiring the necessary skills in pleural ultrasound. Each chapter includes tips for clinical practice and is supplemented by multiple-choice self-assessment questions. The book also covers applications beyond the pleura, ultrasound-guided procedures, training requirements, and equipment information.

On behalf of the authors, we hope this text will help you in the journey of discovering the benefits of pleural ultrasound.

**Claire Tobin**
**Y.C. Gary Lee**

*January 2014*

# Contributors

**Rahul Bhatnagar** MRCP
Clinical Research Fellow,
Southmead Hospital,
Bristol, United Kingdom

**Amelia O. Clive** MRCP
University of Bristol,
Southmead Hospital,
Bristol, United Kingdom

**John Coucher** MB BS MRCP
FRCR FRANZCR
Radiologist,
Princess Alexandra Hospital,
Brisbane, QLD, Australia

**Andreas H. Diacon** MD PhD
Associate Professor,
Division of Medical Physiology,
University of Stellenbosch and
Tygerberg Academic Hospital,
Cape Town, South Africa

**Anthony Edey** MRCP FRCR
Consultant Thoracic Radiologist,
Southmead Hospital,
Bristol, United Kingdom

**James Entwisle** MBBS MRCP
FRCR
Clinical Leader,
Department of Radiology,
Wellington Regional Hospital,
Wellington, New Zealand

**David Feller-Kopman** MD
Director, Bronchoscopy and
Interventional Pulmonology,
and Associate Professor of
Medicine,
Johns Hopkins School of Medicine,
Baltimore, Maryland, USA

**Edward T. Fysh** MB BS BSc
Clinical Research Fellow (Pleural
Diseases) and Senior Registrar
(Intensive Care),
Pleural Diseases Unit,
Sir Charles Gairdner Hospital,
Perth, WA, Australia

**Luke Garske** MB BS FRACP
Respiratory Physician,
Department of Respiratory
Medicine,
Princess Alexandra Hospital,
Brisbane, QLD, Australia

**Christopher Gilbert** DO
Department of Pulmonary
and Critical Care Medicine,
Interventional Pulmonary,
Johns Hopkins School of Medicine,
Baltimore, Maryland, USA

**Rob Hallifax** BM BCh (Oxon)
MA (Cantab) MRCP
Oxford Pleural Unit and Oxford
Centre for Respiratory Medicine,
Churchill Hospital,
Oxford, United Kingdom

**Y. C. Gary Lee** MBChB PhD FCCP
FRACP
Consultant and Director of Pleural
Services,
Department of Respiratory
Medicine,
Sir Charles Gairdner Hospital,
Perth, WA, Australia
*and*
Winthrop Professor of Respiratory
Medicine,
Centre for Asthma, Allergy and
Respiratory Research,
School of Medicine and
Pharmacology,
University of Western Australia,
Perth, WA, Australia

**Scott King**
Chief Sonographer,
Princess Alexandra Hospital,
Brisbane, QLD, Australia

**Coenraad F. N. Koegelenberg**
MBChB, FCP, MRCP, PhD
Senior Specialist,
Division of Pulmonology,
University of Stellenbosch and
Tygerberg Academic Hospital,
Cape Town, South Africa

**Nick A. Maskell** DM FRCP
Consultant Respiratory Physician
   and Senior Lecturer,
Academic Lung Unit,
School of Clinical Sciences,
Learning and Research Centre,
University of Bristol,
Southmead Hospital,
Bristol, United Kingdom

**Sam Phillips** MBChB FACEM
Emergency Consultant,
Sir Charles Gairdner Hospital,
Perth, WA, Australia

**Nagmi R. Qureshi** BSc MBBS
   MRCP FRCR
Consultant Radiologist,
Department of Radiology,
Papworth Hospital,
Cambridgeshire, United Kingdom

**Najib M. Rahman** BM BCh
   MA (Oxon) MRCP (UK) MSc
   (LSHTM) D PHil
Academic Clinical Lecturer,
Oxford Pleural Unit and Oxford
   Centre for Respiratory Medicine,
Churchill Hospital,
Oxford, United Kingdom

**James Rippey** MBBS DDU DCH
   FACEM
Emergency Consultant,
University of Western Australia
*and*
Sir Charles Gairdner Hospital
*and*
King Edward Memorial Hospital
   for Women,
Perth, WA, Australia

**Nicola Smith** BHB MBChB
   FRACP
Consultant in Respiratory and
   General Medicine,
Department of Respiratory
   Medicine,
Wellington Regional Hospital,
Wellington, New Zealand

**Sze K. Tan** MBBS MMed
Department of General Medicine,
Khoo Teck Puat Hospital,
Singapore
*and*
Department of Respiratory
   Medicine,
Sir Charles Gairdner Hospital,
Perth, WA, Australia

**Claire L. Tobin** BA BMBCh MRCP
Clinical Pleural Fellow,
Department of Respiratory
   Medicine,
Sir Charles Gairdner Hospital,
Perth, WA, Australia

**John M. Wrightson** MA MB BChir
   MRCP
Clinical Research Fellow,
Oxford Pleural Unit,
Oxford NIHR Biomedical Research
   Centre,
University of Oxford,
Oxford, United Kingdom

# Clinical Indications for Pleural Ultrasound

Sze K. Tan and Y.C. Gary Lee

## INTRODUCTION

Pleural disease is commonly encountered in clinical practice. An estimated 3000 people per million population each year develop a pleural effusion.[1] The United States alone sees an estimated 1.5 million cases of pleural effusions annually.[2]

Clinical workup of a pleural effusion inevitably involves radiologic imaging techniques that may include chest radiography, ultrasonograpy, computed tomography, and magnetic resonance imaging or positron emission tomography. Sampling of the pleural fluid or tissue is often required in the management of pleural effusions. A safe and cost-effective approach is therefore essential in the diagnostic workup of these patients.

## ADVANTAGES OF PLEURAL ULTRASOUND OVER CLINICAL ASSESSMENT AND CHEST RADIOGRAPHY

The growing availability of relatively inexpensive and portable ultrasound machines has greatly enhanced the diagnostic capabilities of clinicians in the assessment of pleural diseases. Pleural ultrasound offers significant advantages in the detection of pleural effusion, estimating the size and nature of the effusion, and identifying loculations and relations with other vital structures. Ultrasonography provides prompt, accurate, radiation-free, real-time point-of-care imaging. Pleural ultrasound performs better than chest radiographs and is comparable to computed tomography (CT) scans in the assessment of pleural diseases in ambulatory and critically ill patients.[3,4] The portable nature of modern ultrasound machines allows easy bedside examinations and contributes to its growing popularity.

A rapidly growing number of centers employ ultrasonography before all pleural procedures to enhance procedural safety. The critical role of pleural ultrasound in improving the accuracy and safety of pleural puncture sites has been well established in multiple reports.[5–9] Diacon et al. have shown that even in "expert hands" the determination of the presence of pleural effusion based on physical examination and chest x-ray (CXR) was inaccurate, with an alarming 15% error rate. Without the use of ultrasound, 10% of patients will suffer accidental organ puncture to the lung, spleen, or liver during attempted thoracentesis[6] (Figures 1.1–1.3). Hirsch *et al.* reported that ultrasound-guided thoracentesis was successful in 87% of patients who had failed an attempted aspiration guided by physical examination and chest radiography.[5] These findings herald a need for change to the mandatory use of ultrasonography in localizing a safe and accurate site for thoracentesis.

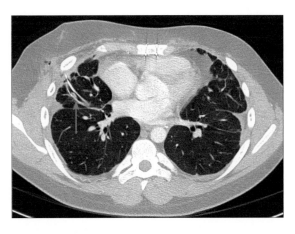

**Figure 1.1** Chest drain (arrow) inserted into the right lung. Unfortunately, this patient had received a lung transplant.

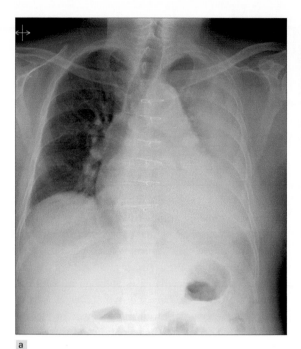

a

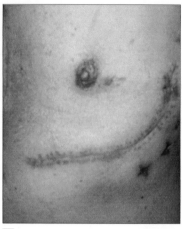

b

**Figure 1.2** Puncture of the left ventricle (LV) during non-ultrasound-guided chest drain insertion in a patient post-CABG with left pleural effusion. (a) CXR preprocedure. (b) Urgent cardiothoracic surgery for extensive LV repair was required. (Photo courtesy of Dr Helen Ward.)

Clinical signs of a pleural effusion may be mimicked by other pulmonary conditions, such as consolidation, collapse, and an elevated hemidiaphragm. Signs of an underlying pleural effusion cannot be differentiated from those of an underlying liver or spleen. A preprocedural ultrasound in these cases is therefore necessary to distinguish between these conditions and to select an appropriate site for thoracentesis.[10]

Chest radiographs are not as sensitive as ultrasound in detecting pleural fluid and may appear normal in such cases. As much as 500 ml of pleural fluid may be present without blunting of the lateral costophrenic angle,[11] and large effusions may be missed on a supine radiograph, as the pleural fluid layers posteriorly.[12] A loculated pleural effusion, on the other hand, may occasionally be mistaken for a solid tumor on chest radiograph. Ultrasound can separate fluid from both consolidation and atelectasis. Pleural ultrasound thus improves the yield and safety of thoracentesis in effusions, particularly in small or complex collections.[6,7,13]

## PLEURAL ULTRASONOGRAPHY BY CHEST PHYSICIANS

### Diagnostic competencies

Physicians given appropriate training can perform pleural ultrasound to a standard comparable with thoracic specialist radiologists. In a UK study,[14] physician-delivered thoracic ultrasound was accurate and had a high level of agreement (99.6% for detection of pleural fluid and 89.3% for assessing technical feasibility of pleural fluid for aspiration) with specialist thoracic radiologists.

### Procedural competencies

The benefits of preprocedural pleural ultrasound are equally applicable whether the ultrasound examination was performed by radiologists or chest physicians.[8,9] In a prospective study of 941 thoracenteses by interventional radiologists under ultrasound guidance in a tertiary referral hospital, the incidence of postprocedural pneumothorax was 2.5%, with only 0.8% requiring tube thoracostomies. These figures compare favorably with the incidence of complications previously reported in the literature for thoracenteses without direct imaging guidance.[8] Similarly, a study of pulmonologists in Mayo Clinic[9] showed that a

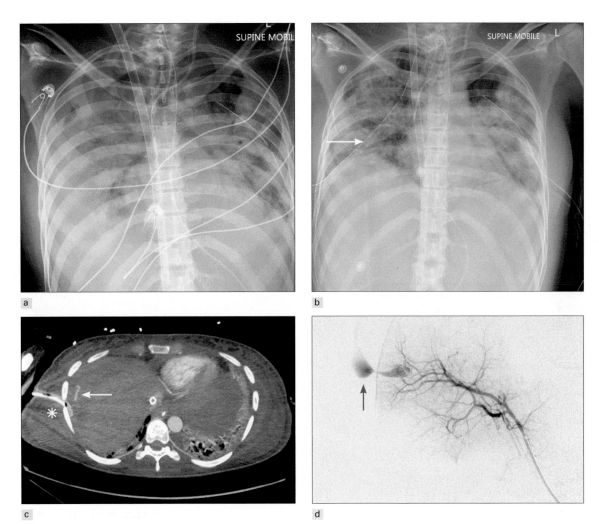

**Figure 1.3** Hemoperitoneum caused by chest drain insertion. (a) CXR prior to right-sided chest drain insertion in a patient with bilateral pneumonia and pleural effusions. (b) CXR post-drain insertion (arrow). (c) CT angiogram illustrating entry site of chest drain (asterisk) and active bleeding (arrow) from trauma to the adjacent liver during insertion. (d) Arterial extravasation of contrast pre-embolization (arrow).

comprehensive teaching program and compulsory use of ultrasound before thoracentesis significantly reduced the incidence of post-procedural pneumothorax from 8.6% to 1.1%. The need for tube thoracostomy drainage of pneumothorax dropped from 6% to 0%. This occurred despite an increase in the number of thoracenteses performed by the physicians. This holds true even in the intensive care unit, where the pneumothorax rate after ultrasound-guided thoracentesis in patients receiving mechanical ventilation was 1.2%.[9] Therefore, appropriately trained physicians can achieve comparable results to those of radiologists.

## Recommendations

Competency in ultrasonography depends on training, and various training guidelines are now available. Many professional medical bodies have also issued statements regarding the role of ultrasonography by clinicians in the management of pleural diseases.

The British Thoracic Society pleural disease guidelines in 2010 strongly recommended the use of thoracic ultrasound guidance for all pleural procedures.[15] This is especially important when aspirating small or loculated pleural effusions, where there is near or complete opacity of the hemithorax, but without contralateral mediastinal shift, or after an unsuccessful attempt of

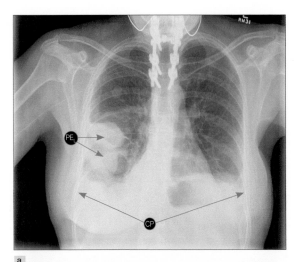

a

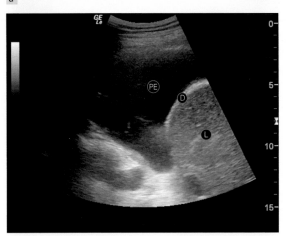

b

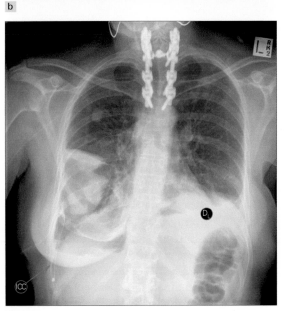

c

aspiration without imaging guidance. It has been proposed that at least level 1 competency according to the Royal College of Radiologist guidelines (www.rcr.ac.uk/docs/radiology/pdf/ultrasound.pdf) is required to safely and effectively perform thoracic ultrasound independently.

The Australasian Society for Ultrasound in Medicine similarly supports the use of ultrasonography by medical specialists, other than radiologists or sonographers, who have undergone appropriate training and credentialing.[16] Various levels of credentialing have been cited (see www.asum.com.au) and serve as a guide to the level of competency expected of clinicians utilizing ultrasound in clinical practice. The Critical Care Network of the American College of Chest Physicians, together with La Société de Réanimation de Langue Française, has defined in its consensus statement the specific skill sets required of intensivists and chest physicians involved with pleural ultrasonography. Also included are other aspects of critical care ultrasonography.[17] Specific training requirements stipulated by the above medical bodies are detailed in Chapter 11.

## DIAGNOSTIC APPLICATIONS OF PLEURAL ULTRASOUND

### Detection of pleural fluid

Pleural ultrasound is a sensitive modality for detecting pleural effusions, with a diagnostic accuracy of more than 90%,[3,4,14] and is significantly superior to chest radiography[3,4,18] (Figures 1.4 and 1.5). Pleural fluid is easily visualized by its characteristic appearance on ultrasound.[19,20] Typically, it is seen as an echo-free or dark zone that changes its shape with respiratory movements or contains movable echo densities. Ultrasound can confirm the presence of pleural fluid, especially in small or loculated pleural effusions, and distinguish it from pleural thickening[21] (see also Chapter 5).

**Figure 1.4** A patient with an elevated left hemidiaphragm, where the presence and extent of a right pleural effusion may be underestimated on a routine chest radiograph. (a) CXR showing multiple right pleural fluid loculations (PE$_L$) and bilateral blunting of costophrenic angles (CP). (b) Ultrasound demonstrating the moderate pleural effusion (PE) as well as liver (L) and diaphragm (D). (c) CXR post-insertion of a right intercostal catheter (ICC). The elevated left hemi-diaphragm (D$_L$) may lead one to underestimate the extent of the right effusion on the initial CXR.

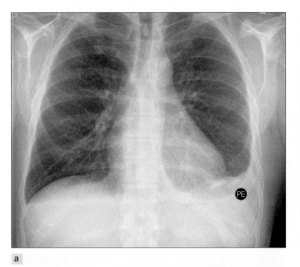

a

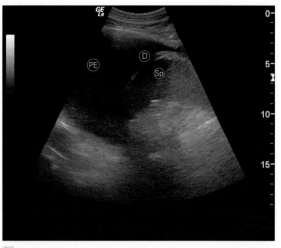

b

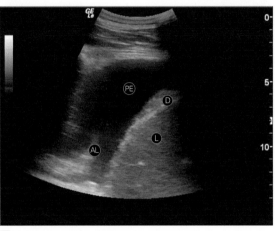

c

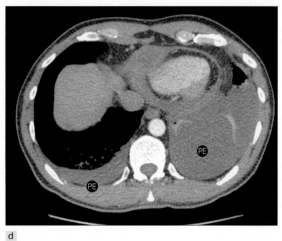

d

## Quantification of pleural fluid

Pleural ultrasound gives a better estimate of the volume of pleural fluid than a chest radiograph.[18] This was especially evident when the sonographic estimation of pleural fluid volume in a supine patient was compared with a lateral decubitus chest radiograph.[18] There are various methods of estimating the volume of pleural fluid with ultrasound; both qualitative[14,22,23] and quantitative[24–27] means have been described. Estimating the fluid volume may aid in determining the safety and need for thoracentesis,[25,26] and assessing the depth of pleural fluid from the chest wall will guide the degree of penetration required for safe thoracentesis.

**Figure 1.5** A patient with bilateral pleural effusions that are not fully appreciated on a routine chest radiograph. (a) The chest radiograph demonstrates only a left pleural effusion (PE). (b) Ultrasound of the left hemithorax confirming a moderate left pleural effusion (PE) (D = diaphragm, Sp = spleen). (c) Ultrasound also demonstrates a right pleural effusion (PE) in the same patient, not apparent on the CXR ( AL = atelectatic lung, L = liver, D = diaphragm). (d) A CT thorax confirming the presence of bilateral pleural effusions (PE).

## Nature of pleural fluid

The sonographic findings of the pleural fluid often help to determine the nature of the pleural effusion. Four basic patterns of internal echogenicity of pleural fluid have been described: anechoic, complex non-septated, complex septated, and homogeneously echogenic[28] (see Chapter 5). The relationship between these patterns and their nature, i.e., whether it is a transudative or an exudative effusion, has been well described in various studies.[5,10,28,29] Other associated features seen on ultrasound, such as thickened pleura, lung parenchymal lesions, pleural and diaphragmatic nodules, and diaphragmatic thickening, are also helpful in providing further insight into the nature of the pleural effusion.[28,29]

## Pleural loculations and adhesions

Pleural ultrasound allows better characterization of pleural fluid collections, with fibrin strands, septations, and loculations more readily detected on ultrasonography than on CT scans[6,30] (Figure 1.6).

The patterns of echogenicity and presence of septation or loculation may influence the subsequent approach to management. In the study by Tu et al.,[31] the presence of septations and the increasing echogenicity of the pleural fluid suggested a higher likelihood of empyema, and hence the need for diagnostic thoracentesis and probable chest tube insertion.

The efficacy of image-guided percutaneous drainage of thoracic empyema can also be predicted by the preprocedural sonographic patterns. The chances of success were better with either an anechoic or complex nonseptated rather than a complex septated empyema.[32] This has led some authors to suggest that patients with empyema should receive a thoracic ultrasound early and be stratified according to the sonographic appearance. Depending on the severity of septations on ultrasound, mechanical adhesiolysis via thoracoscopy or thoracotomy may be required early on for optimal treatment.[33] This approach has yet to be formally tested but highlights the potential contribution of ultrasonography to conventional diagnostic or management algorithms.

Pleural ultrasound enables the detection of pleural adhesions and can provide useful information before thoracosopic procedures.[19,34] A preprocedural pleural ultrasound potentially reduces complications by guiding trocar placement and helps determine the need for open thoracotomy in patients who are planned for video-assisted thoracoscopic surgery. Similarly, pleural ultrasound before medical thoracoscopy may help to select an optimal site for pleural access and thus reduce pleural access failure rates.[35]

## Recognizing features of malignant pleural effusions

Pleural ultrasound can provide useful clues toward the diagnosis of malignant pleural effusion.[36,37] In the study by Qureshi *et al.*, pleural ultrasound is able to distinguish malignant from benign effusions with an overall sensitivity of 79% and specificity of 100%; these figures are comparable to those of contrast-enhanced CT scanning.[36] Ultrasound can detect thickening and nodularity of the parietal, visceral, and diaphragmatic pleura, as well as demonstrate loss of the five diaphragmatic layers (see Chapter 6)—all are features that suggest a malignant pleural effusion in the absence of empyema. Pleural ultrasound is more sensitive than contrast-enhanced CT scans in demonstrating visceral pleural disease and diaphragmatic nodularity[36] (Figure 1.7).

Pleural and chest wall invasion by lung cancer may also be evaluated with thoracic ultrasound (see Chapter 10). High-frequency ultrasound can help distinguish the tumor from other soft tissues of the chest wall and pleura.[38] The information obtained helps to determine the resectability of the tumor as well as the site and extent of resection. This has important implications with regard to patient management and prognostication.

The shape and movement of the diaphragm can also be assessed.[19] Diaphragmatic palsy, e.g., from tumor infiltration of the phrenic nerve, may be diagnosed by real-time visualization on ultrasound, and can influence management.

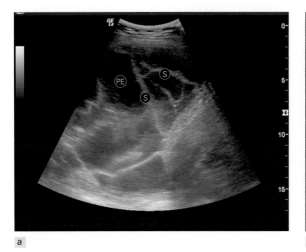

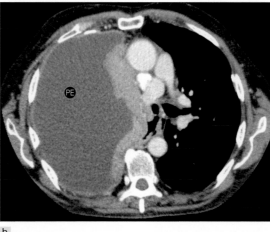

a                                                                    b

**Figure 1.6** A patient with a right malignant pleural effusion. (a) Multiple septations (S) in pleural effusion (PE) are easily seen on pleural ultrasonography. (b) CT thorax of the same patient with no evidence of septations (PE = pleural effusion).

**Figure 1.7** Pleural nodularity (PN) and diaphragmatic thickening (D) are easily seen on ultrasonography.

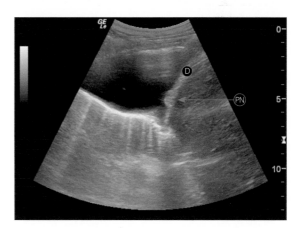

## ULTRASONOGRAPHY IN PLEURAL PROCEDURES

In addition to thoracentesis, pleural ultrasound can guide other pleural interventions, such as chest drain insertions and transthoracic biopsies[19,39] (see Chapters 9 and 10). Ultrasound guidance has been used effectively in chest drain insertion to evacuate different types of pleural effusions.[32,39,40] Accuracy of tube placement and procedural safety are significantly enhanced by pleural ultrasonography. Real-time imaging can also allow the operator to monitor the adequacy of drainage during the procedure.[39]

Thoracic ultrasound has been used to guide biopsies of pleura, peripheral lung lesions, chest wall, and mediastinal lesions.[41–45] Ultrasound-guided pleural biopsy has been shown to have a higher diagnostic sensitivity for pleural tuberculosis and pleural malignancies over the traditional "blind" Abrams needle biopsies.[41] Ultrasound can help localize peripheral lung lesions and guide biopsies under real time.[42–44] Diagnostic yields of up to 77% have been obtained for subpleural lung nodules less than 2 cm in diameter.[43] Success rates up to 96% for biopsying transthoracic lesions less than 3 cm in diameter have been reported.[45]

Being able to observe accurately the course of the biopsy needle in real-time imaging also reduces the risks of lung puncture and post-procedural pneumothorax.[42–45] Similarly, large vessels may be avoided during needle biopsies.[19] Other advantages of ultrasound guidance include a shorter procedure time[42,44] and the ability to screen for pneumothorax immediately post-biopsy[19] (see Chapter 7).

Ultrasound-assisted cutting needle biopsy has been proven safe even when performed by chest physicians for small (<2 cm) lung lesions abutting or involving the pleura.[46] In this study by Diacon et al., the sensitivity of the biopsy for neoplastic disease was 85.5% (and 100% for malignant mesothelioma). The rate of pneumothorax was 4%, of which only half required pleural drainage.

## CONCLUSION

Pleural ultrasound has firmly established its place in the diagnostic workup of pleural diseases. It can accurately identify the presence of pleural fluid, pleural adhesions and loculations, and features suggestive of pleural malignancies. Valuable information of other thoracic structures, e.g., the diaphragm and the chest wall, can be gained and may guide subsequent therapy. The benefits in improving procedural safety make pleural ultrasound an indispensable tool for all pleural procedures. This benefit is independent of the specialty of the operator. Pleural ultrasound has become mandatory before all pleural procedures in a growing number of centers, and adequate training is paramount to fully realize its advantages.

## REFERENCES

1. Light RW, Lee YC. *Textbook of pleural diseases*, 2nd ed. Arnold Hodder, London, 2008.

2. Sahn SA. The value of pleural fluid analysis. *Am J Med Sci* 2008; 335: 7–15.

3. Zanobetti M, Poggioni C, Pini R. Can chest ultrasonography replace chest radiography for evaluation of acute dyspnoea in the ED? *Chest* 2011; 139: 1140–1147.

4. Xirouchaki N, Magkanas E, Vaporidi K, et al. Lung ultrasound in critically ill patients: comparison with bedside chest radiography. *Intensive Care Med* 2011; 37: 1488–1493.

5. Hirsch JH, Rogers JV, Mack LA. Real-time sonography of pleural opacities. *AJR Am J Roentgenol* 1981; 136: 297–301.

6. Diacon AH, Brutsche MH, Soler M. Accuracy of pleural puncture sites. A prospective comparison of clinical examination with ultrasound. *Chest* 2003; 123: 436–441.

7. Ravin CE. Thoracocentesis of loculated pleural effusions using grey scale ultrasonic guidance. *Chest* 1977; 71: 686–688.

8. Jones PW, Moyers JP, Rogers JT, et al. Ultrasound guided thoracentesis: is it a safer method? *Chest* 2003; 123: 418–423.

9. Duncan DR, Morgenthaler TL, Ryu JH, et al. Reducing iatrogenic risk in thoracentesis. *Chest* 2009; 135: 1315–1320.

10. McLoud TC, Flower CDR. Imaging the pleura: sonography, CT and MR imaging. *AJR Am J Roentgenol* 1991; 156: 1145–1153

11. Blackmore CC, Black WC, Dallas RV, et al. Pleural fluid volume estimation: a chest radiograph prediction rule. *Acad Radiol* 1996; 3: 103–109.

12. Mueller NL. Imaging of the pleural. *Radiology* 1993; 186: 297–309.

13. Weingardt JP, Guico RR, Nemcek AA, et al. Ultrasound findings following failed, clinically directed thoracentesis. *J Clin Ultrasound* 1994; 22: 419–426.

14. Rahman NM, Singanayagam A, Davies HE, et al. Diagnostic accuracy, safety and utilization of respiratory physician-delivered thoracic ultrasound. *Thorax* 2010; 65: 449–453.

15. Havelock T, Teoh R, Laws D, et al. Pleural procedures and thoracic ultrasound: British Thoracic Society pleural disease guideline 2010. *Thorax* 2010; 65 (Suppl 2): ii61–ii76.

16. Australasian Society for Ultrasound in Medicine. Statement on the use of ultrasound by medical practitioners. July 2008. http://www.asum.com.au/site/policies.php (accessed December 21, 2011).

17. Mayo PH, Beaulieu Y, Doelken P, et al. American College of Chest Physicians/La Societe de Reanimation de Langue Francaise statement on competence in critical care ultrasonography. *Chest* 2009; 135: 1050–1060.

18. Eibenberger KL, Dock WI, Ammann ME, et al. Quantifications of pleural effusions: sonography versus radiography. *Radiology* 1994; 191: 681–684.

19. Beckh S, Bolcskei PL, Lessnau K. Real-time chest ultra-sonography: a comprehensive review for the pulmonologist. *Chest* 2002; 122: 1759–1773.

20. Marks WM, Filly RA, Callen PW. Real-time evaluation of pleural lesions: new observations regarding the probability of obtaining free fluid. *Radiology* 1982; 142: 163–164.

21. Wu RG, Yuan A, Liaw YS, et al. Image comparison of real-time gray-scale ultrasound and colour Doppler ultrasound for use in diagnosis of minimal pleural effusion. *Am J Respir Crit Care Med* 1994; 150: 510–514.

22. Medford ARL, Entwisle JJ. Indications for thoracic ultrasound in chest medicine: an observational study. *Postgrad Med J* 2010; 86: 8–11.

23. Tsai TH, Jerng JS, Yang PC. Clinical applications of transthoracic ultrasound in chest medicine. *J Med Ultrasound* 2008; 16: 7–25.

24. Roch A, Bojan M, Michelet P, et al. Usefulness of ultra-sonography in predicting pleural effusions >500ml in patients receiving mechanical ventilation. *Chest* 2005; 127: 224–232.

25. Remerand F, Dellamonica J, Mao Z, et al. Multiplane ultrasound approach to quantify pleural effusion at the bedside. *Intensive Care Med* 2010; 36: 656–664.

26. Usta E, Mustafi M, Zeimer G. Ultrasound estimation of volume of postoperative pleural effusion in cardiac surgery patients. *Interact Cardiovas Thorac Surg* 2010; 10: 204–207.

27. Reuss J. Sonographic imaging of the pleura: nearly 30 years of experience. *Eur J Ultrasound* 1996; 3: 25–39.

28. Yang PC, Luh K, Chang D, et al. Value of sonography in determining the nature of pleural effusion: analysis of 320 cases. *AJR Am J Roentgenol* 1992; 159: 29–33.

29. Sajadieh H, Afzali F, Sajadieh V, et al. Ultrasound as an alternative to aspiration for determining the nature of pleural effusion, especially in older people. *Ann NY Acad Sci* 2004; 1019: 585–592.

30. Heffner JE, Klein JS, Hampson C. Diagnostic utility and clinical application of imaging for pleural space infections. *Chest* 2010; 137: 467–479.

31. Tu CY, Hsu WH, Hsia TC, et al. Pleural effusions in febrile medical ICU patients: chest ultrasound study. *Chest* 2004; 126: 1274–1280.

32. Shankar S, Gulati M, Kang M, et al. Image-guided percutaneous drainage of thoracic empyema: can sonography predict the outcome? *Eur Radiol* 2000; 10: 495–499.

33. Brutsche MH, Tassi G, Gyorik S, et al. Treatment of sonographically stratified multiloculated thoracic empyema by medical thoracoscopy. *Chest* 2005; 128: 3303–3309.

34. Sasaki M, Kawabe M, Hirai S, et al. Preoperative detection of pleural adhesions by chest ultrasonography. *Ann Thorac Surg* 2005; 80: 439–442.

35. Medford ARL, Agrawal S, Bennett JA, et al. Thoracic ultrasound prior to medical thoracoscopy improves pleural access and predicts fibrous septation. *Respirology* 2010; 15: 804–808.

36. Qureshi NR, Rahman NM, Gleeson FV. Thoracic ultrasound in the diagnosis of malignant pleural effusion. *Thorax* 2009; 64: 139–143.

37. Gorg C, Restrepo I, Schwerk WB. Sonography of malignant pleural effusion. *Eur Radiol* 1997; 7: 1195–1198.

38. Sugama Y, Tamaki S, Kitamura S, et al. Ultrasonographic evaluation of pleural and chest wall invasion of lung cancer. *Chest* 1988; 93: 275–279.

39. O'Moore PV, Mueller PR, Simeone JF, et al. Sonographic guidance in diagnostic and therapeutic interventions in the pleural space. *AJR Am J Roentgenol* 1987; 149: 1–5.

40. Liu YH, Lin YC, Liang SJ, et al. Ultrasound-guided pigtail catheters for drainage of various pleural diseases. *Am J Emerg Med* 2010; 28: 915–921.

41. Chang DB, Yang PC, Luh KT, et al. Ultrasound-guided pleural biopsy with tru-cut needle. *Chest* 1991; 100: 1328–1333.

42. Cinti D, Hawkins HB. Aspiration biopsy of peripheral pulmonary masses using real-time sonographic guidance. *AJR Am J Roentgenol* 1984; 142: 1115–1116.

43. Obata K, Ueki J, Dambara T, et al. Repeated ultrasonically guided needle biopsy of small subpleural nodules. *Chest* 1999; 116: 1320–1324.

44. Sheth S, Hamper UM, Stanley DB, et al. US guidance for thoracic biopsy: a valuable alternative to CT. *Radiology* 1999; 210: 721–726.

45. Liao WY, Chen MZ, Chang YL, et al. US-guided transthoracic cutting biopsy for peripheral thoracic lesions less than 3cm in diameter. *Radiology* 2000; 217: 685–691.

46. Diacon AH, Schuurmans MM, Theron J, et al. Safety and yield of ultrasound-assisted transthoracic biopsy performed by pulmonologists. *Respiration* 2004; 71: 519–522.

CHAPTER 1

CHAPTER 1

## MCQ 1

 Which of the following statements are *true* (multiple answers possible)?

a. Pleural ultrasound is superior to a physical examination and chest radiograph in avoiding accidental puncture of visceral organs in pleural procedures.

b. The absence of blunting of the costophrenic angles on chest radiograph reliably excludes the presence of a pleural effusion.

c. A pleural ultrasound should be performed before all pleural procedures, especially if the pleural effusion is small and loculated.

d. Appropriately trained physicians are able to perform pleural ultrasound at a comparable level to specialist thoracic radiologists.

e. The presence of radiation from pleural ultrasonography limits its repeated use in clinical settings.

## MCQ 2

 Which one of the following regarding ultrasound-guided pleural biopsies is *false*?

a. Ultrasound-guided pleural biopsies give better yields than traditional Abrams needle biopsies.

b. Ultrasound-guided biopsies of visualized subpleural lung nodules give higher diagnostic yields than bronchoscopic biopsies.

c. Ultrasound-guided biopsies can be considered in the assessment of peripheral thoracic lesions in patients who are not medically fit to undergo major surgical procedures.

d. Ultrasound-guided biopsies should never be performed for peripheral thoracic lesions less than 3 cm, as the yield is significantly less.

e. Pleural ultrasound may be used to detect post-procedural pneumothoraces.

## MCQ 3

 Pleural ultrasound allows the following:

a. Detection of pleural fluid and its differentiation from solid organs.

b. Better estimation of volume of pleural fluid when compared to a chest radiograph.

c. Differentiation of transudative pleural fluids from exudative ones.

d. Better visualization of pleural thickening and nodularity when compared to other imaging modalities.

e. All of the above.

## MCQ 4

 In addition to the assessment of pleural fluid, pleural ultrasound may also be used in assessing the:

a. Structural features of the diaphragm.

b. Diaphragmatic movements.

c. Pleural and chest wall invasion by lung cancer.

d. Presence of pleural adhesions.

e. All of the above.

## ANSWERS

 **1.** a, c, and d are all true.

Pleural fluid may be detected on ultrasound and not visualized on CXR (see Chapter 1). Ultrasound is radiation-free.

 **2.** d  See Chapter 1 for reference.

 **3.** e

 **4.** e

# Basic Physics of Diagnostic Ultrasound and Control "Knobology"

Nagmi R. Qureshi

## INTRODUCTION

This chapter provides an introduction to the basic physics of diagnostic ultrasound. A clear understanding of the principles of ultrasound is vital for appreciating the potential limitations of thoracic ultrasound and interpreting commonly encountered artifacts. The function of the main ultrasound controls will be discussed, and how these can be adjusted to optimize the ultrasound settings to ensure a diagnostic quality image is routinely obtained.

## GENERATION AND TRANSMISSION OF THE ULTRASOUND WAVE

Ultrasound is a sound wave with frequencies that range from 2 to 20 MHz. These frequencies are much greater than sound waves audible to the human ear, which range from 20 Hz to 20 kHz.

Ultrasound waves are produced by piezoelectric crystal elements within a transducer. This crystal has the ability to change shape and thickness when an electrical voltage is applied across it, causing it to vibrate at a specific range of frequencies that produces a sound wave. Transducers consist of multiple elements that are usually pulsed sequentially and function as both the transmitter of sound and the receiver of the reflected echo. As each element cannot simultaneously transmit and receive an echo, another sound wave cannot be generated until the initial echo has been received. The sound waves from the ultrasound beam are transmitted as a series of longitudinal waves that vibrate back and forth, producing a wave of compression and rarefaction of the surrounding tissues. Each repetition of this back-and-forth motion produces a new wave, the length of which represents its wavelength. Unlike x-rays, a sound wave requires a medium for transmission. Because

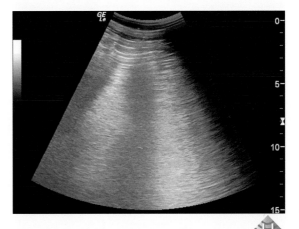

**Figure 2.1** Curvilinear transducer that shows no transmission of the ultrasound wave until gel is applied to the transducer face. View E-book for ultrasound clip or watch it at http://goo.gl/ZadCSC.

of the difference in the acoustic impedance (effectively, the fraction of the ultrasound wave transmitted or reflected) between the probe and air, a coupling medium, gel, is used to help match their impedances and enable through-transmission of the ultrasound wave (Figure 2.1—clip).

The speed of transmission of ultrasound is independent of its frequency and depends on the density and compressibility of the tissue through which it is traveling. For practical purposes, all tissues except bone and air have an average velocity of 1540 m/s. Solids and liquids typically consist of tight, large particles, are less compressible, and transmit sound rapidly. Air, however, is a poor transmitter of sound due to its low density and high compressibility.[1]

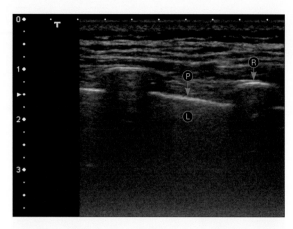

**Figure 2.2** Pleural ultrasound showing echogenic reflection of the ultrasound wave from the rib (R) and pleural–lung interface. P = pleura, L = lung.

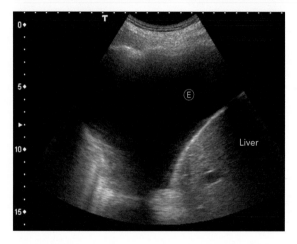

**Figure 2.3** Normal appearance of a simple pleural effusion (E) that appears as an echo-poor space. This is due to limited reflection and attenuation of the ultrasound wave by fluid.

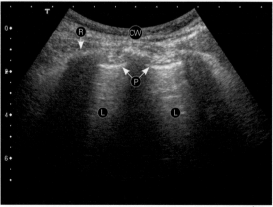

# INTERACTION OF SOUND WAVES WITH MATTER

As an ultrasound wave passes through matter it interacts in several different ways and can be reflected, transmitted forward, absorbed, scattered, or refracted.

## Reflection

The ultrasound image is produced from the proportion of the transmitted beam that is reflected back to the transducer. The amount reflected at an interface is primarily dependent on the difference in the acoustic impedance of the adjacent tissues. This is defined as the product of the density and velocity of sound in the material. The greater the difference in impedance at an interface, the greater the proportion of the echo that is reflected back and the stronger and brighter the echo displayed. Highly reflective interfaces cause strong echoes that are displayed as a bright spot on the screen. This is typically seen at bone and air interfaces where nearly 99% of the wave can be reflected, leaving only 1% to be transmitted forward (Figure 2.2). The opposite is seen with poorly reflective interfaces such as fluid, where there is little or no reflection, and this is displayed as an echo-poor area (Figure 2.3). In addition, the angle of the incident wave can also influence the echo. Typically the closer the transmitted wave is to the perpendicular, the stronger the echo.

## Attenuation

As the wave travels forward, it continuously loses energy and intensity, with fewer echoes being reflected back at each interface. This is generally referred to as attenuation and primarily occurs due to absorption and, to a lesser extent, scatter. The degree of attenuation or the attenuation coefficient is dependent upon the density of the material and the frequency of the transducer. Typically water produces the least attenuation and provides an excellent acoustic window for scanning. Bone and lung have the highest attenuation coefficients and are poor transmitters of ultrasound (Figure 2.4—clip). Attenuation can lead to artifacts, which will be discussed later in this section.

**Figure 2.4** Normal ultrasound appearance of the lung (L), pleura (P), and ribs (R). CW = chest wall. There is poor transmission of the ultrasound wave into the normally aerated lung seen below the pleural line (in between rib shadowing). View E-book for ultrasound clip or watch it at http://goo.gl/quO9GC.

## Absorption

Absorption involves the conversion of the ultrasound wave into thermal energy. Tissue absorption usually increases with higher frequencies, resulting in poorer penetration, and is the reason why high-frequency probes are used to image structures close to the probe, such as the thyroid, testes, and the pleural surface.

## Scattering

Scattering occurs when the sound wave encounters microscopic structures that are much smaller than its wavelength, with little or no direct reflection back, causing the sound wave to be radiated in all directions. This may result in speculation of the ultrasound image—multiple bright echoes on the screen.

## Refraction

Refraction refers to the bending of the ultrasound wave as it travels from one tissue to the next. This causes the sound wave to slow down. As the frequency of the wave remains the same, the wavelength changes to accommodate the change in velocity, causing the beam to change direction. This can produce "edge shadowing" artifacts, which will be discussed later.

## FORMATION OF THE ULTRASOUND IMAGE

The grayscale ultrasound image is constructed from the echoes transmitted back to the transducer. Each echo is displayed as a point that corresponds to its position in the body. This is determined by the time taken and strength of the echo to return to the transducer, which corresponds to the depth of the interface producing the echo. The energy from the returning echoes causes the transducer elements to change shape, inducing a voltage change between the transducer electrodes. This voltage is amplified and entered along the corresponding scan line in memory locations that correspond to where the echoes have arisen, and these are digitally displayed on the ultrasound screen.[2]

## CHARACTERISTICS OF THE ULTRASOUND BEAM

The ultrasound beam is typically divided into a near (Fresnel) and far (Fraunhofer) zone, with the intensity of the sound wave varying along its length and width. The intensity of the beam is strongest and most focused in the near zone, which allows for better spatial resolution. Beyond this the beam starts to diverge and become less intense and useful. Optimal ultrasound imaging therefore occurs in the near zone. The depth of the near zone is determined by the diameter of the transducer and the frequency of the ultrasound. It can be increased by using larger-diameter and higher-frequency transducers.

Although using a high-frequency ultrasound beam can improve resolution, they are limited by their depth of penetration. This is primarily related to increased tissue absorption with increased frequency. In everyday scanning the decision as to the most appropriate transducer frequency range to use is usually a compromise between good image resolution and adequate depth of penetration (Figures 2.5a and b).

CHAPTER 2

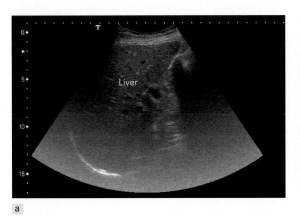

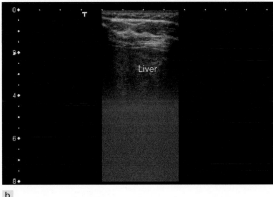

a    b

**Figure 2.5** Upper abdominal ultrasound performed using (a) curvilinear transducer that allows the full depth of the liver to be scanned and (b) linear transducer that only allows the superficial aspect to be imaged, with poor depth penetration.

## TRANSDUCERS

Most ultrasound machines have specific presets that can be used for thoracic ultrasound imaging. The musculoskeletal or thyroid preset can be used for visualizing the pleura, whereas the abdominal preset is routinely used for assessing pleural effusions and parenchymal pathology.

Linear transducers usually operate with high frequencies that range from 7 to 12 MHz. They produce a rectangular field of view that allows optimal spatial resolution in the superficial zone. Therefore, they are mainly used for assessing superficial structures, e.g., the chest wall, pleura, subcutaneous tissues, and lymph nodes (Figure 2.6).

Curvilinear transducers produce a wide, fan-shaped field of view and operate at lower frequencies in the range of 2–6 MHz. Lower frequencies allow better depth of penetration, but at the expense of poorer resolution. Curvilinear transducers are used for imaging deeper structures, e.g., pleural effusions, upper abdominal organs, and mediastinal structures, and they are also helpful in more obese patients (Figure 2.7).

Sector transducers are typically used in echocardiography; however, they can be useful for thoracic imaging in thinner patients when access is difficult, e.g., narrow intercostal spaces. They operate in a frequency range of 1–3 MHz and provide a small field of view near the skin with a wider field of view at depth, and therefore good depth penetration. However, at low frequencies images can appear grainy.

## ARTIFACTS

Artifacts can be helpful and allow better characterization of pathological processes, or a hindrance by obscuring and degrading the image quality. In this section, we describe the artifacts that are commonly encountered during a thoracic and upper abdominal ultrasound examination and their mechanism of formation.

### Reverberation artifact

This artifact occurs when there is a significant difference in the acoustic impedance at a tissue interface. It is most commonly seen at soft tissue–air or soft tissue–bone interfaces. As these interfaces are strong reflectors, the echo reflected back to an adjacent interface or the transducer is re-reflected back and forth. At the pleura–lung interface, this gives the spurious appearance of a series of multiple adjacent regularly spaced echogenic parallel lines below the pleural line (Figure 2.8—clip and Figure 2.9).

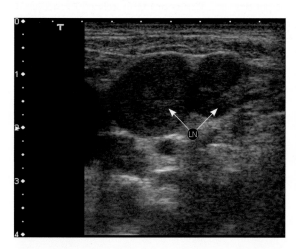

**Figure 2.6** Neck ultrasound demonstrating two pathological lymph nodes (LN) performed using a linear 11 MHz high-frequency transducer. This shows good image resolution within the near field to a depth of 2 cm.

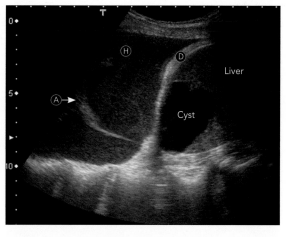

**Figure 2.7** Thoracic ultrasound performed using a curvilinear 6 MHz low-frequency transducer. This allows good penetration and resolution to a depth of 10 cm and demonstrates a diffusely echogenic hemothorax (H) and compressive atelectasis (A). This acts as a good acoustic window, allowing the hemidiaphragm (D) and liver to be nicely visualized.

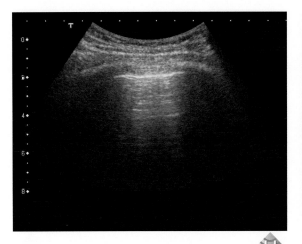

**Figure 2.8** Reverberation artifact. Pleural ultrasound performed using a linear high-frequency transducer that shows the lung sliding back and forth with normal respiration. Behind the echogenic pleural line, which is seen 2 cm from the skin surface, are multiple horizontal echogenic "reverberating" lines. View E-book for ultrasound clip or watch it at http://goo.gl/Arw5Xz.

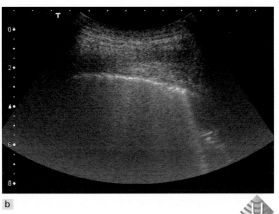

**Figure 2.9** Reverberation artifact. Pleural ultrasound demonstrating the multiple parallel echogenic lines (white arrows). Adjacent rib shadowing (blue arrow) is also noted.

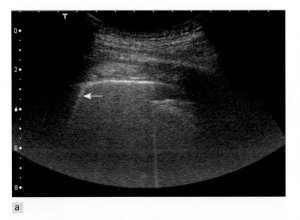

a          b

**Figure 2.10** Comet-tail artifact. (a) Thoracic ultrasound of the left costophrenic angle demonstrating the tapering vertical echogenic "comet tail" line (arrow) that is seen with normal lung excursion. (b) Ultrasound clip of comet-tail artifact. View E-book for ultrasound clip or watch it at http://goo.gl/IKLl65.

## Comet-tail artifact

This is a form of reverberation artifact that appears as a trail of dense continuous tapering echogenic lines that merge to simulate a comet tail (Figure 2.10a and b—clip). It is usually seen when the reflective interfaces are closely spaced. It is commonly seen at the pleura–lung interface at the costophrenic angles or with metallic objects such as surgical clips and cholesterol foci. Generally the greater the difference in acoustic impedance between the interfaces, or smaller the object size, the stronger the echogenicity of the artifact.

CHAPTER 2

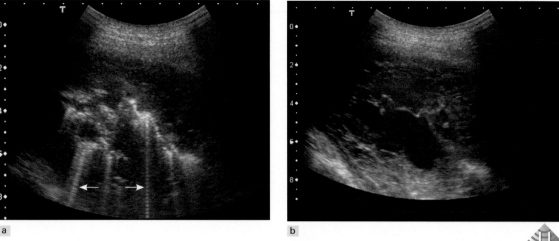

a b

**Figure 2.11** Ring-down artifact. (a) Thoracic ultrasound showing pleural thickening and a complex effusion in a patient with mesothelioma. There are numerous echogenic "ringing" gas bubbles causing a series of small, discrete parallel echogenic lines (arrows). (b) Ultrasound clip. View E-book for ultrasound clip or watch it at http://goo.gl/TD6xsX.

## Ring-down artifact

This artifact is usually seen with gas collections or air bubbles. It is produced when the transmitted ultrasound energy causes the adjacent air bubble to resonate or "ring." These vibrations create a continuous sound wave that is transmitted back to the transducer. Because this continuous sound wave is emitted after the transducer receives the initial reflection, the ultrasound system perceives the emitted sound as coming from structures deeper in the body. These artifacts appear as a solid series of small parallel echogenic bands radiating away from the gas collection[3] (Figure 2.11a and b—clip). This artifact can also be seen when imaging the liver, where it appears as multiple, vertical, long, narrow bands or lines extending down from the posterior surface of the right hemidiaphragm.

## Mirroring artifact

Mirroring occurs when sound waves are reflected from a curved, strong, reflective surface. At this surface the sound wave can scatter and be reflected by an adjacent part of the curved surface. This increases the time taken for the echo to return to the transducer and is interpreted as a reflecting interface that is deeper to the curved surface than is in fact the case.[4] In thoracic ultrasound this is usually seen with the diaphragm, where the liver or spleen can appear to lie in the lung (Figure 2.12) (also see Chapter 4, Figure 4.28). Knowledge of this

artifact is important when imaging the lower thorax as the liver, and adjacent ascites, if mirrored, can falsely suggest the presence of parenchymal consolidation (parenchymal hepatization) and an adjacent effusion. Mirroring is most commonly seen when imaging thin patients and can be overcome by using a higher-frequency transducer.

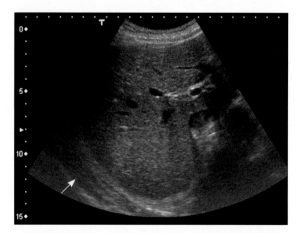

**Figure 2.12** Mirroring artifact. The lung–diaphragm interface behaves as a strong reflector and gives the spurious appearance of the liver (arrow) lying deep to the hemidiaphragm and within the lung.

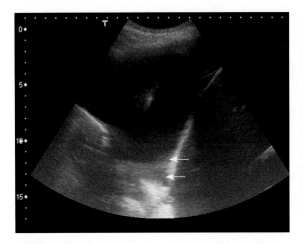

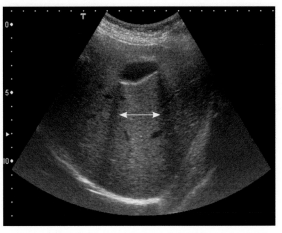

**Figure 2.13** Side-lobe artifact. Echo-poor simple pleural effusion, with side-lobe artifacts simulating septations and dependent debris (white arrows). This is due to the highly reflective fluid-lung interface.

**Figure 2.14** Refractive artifact. Normal appearance of the gallbladder, with shadowing radiating from the edges (arrow).

## Side-lobe artifact

Side lobes occur due to vibrations that arise from the edge of the transducer. These produce low-intensity ultrasound waves that lie obliquely outside the main beam. As the transducer cannot discriminate between echoes generated by the side lobes and those from the main beam, they appear as artifactual echoes within the main beam. This artifact is usually seen near strong, curved, highly reflective surfaces such as the diaphragm, or near fluid-filled/large cystic structures, e.g., pleural effusions or the bladder. This artifact can give the erroneous appearance of sludge or debris within the cystic structure (Figure 2.13). The artifact can be overcome by repositioning the transducer.

## Edge-shadowing/refractive artifact

This artifact occurs when the ultrasound beam strikes the edge of a rounded structure and is reflected at an angle. This causes fewer echoes to be reflected straight back to the transducer, and is perceived as a shadow arising from the edge (Figure 2.14).

## Acoustic or posterior enhancement

Acoustic enhancement is seen when a sound wave travels through a poorly attenuating medium with little or no reflection. This allows more of the ultrasound wave to be transmitted forward with stronger echoes and posterior enhancement immediately beyond it. This is usually indicative of a fluid structure, e.g., simple cyst, gallbladder, and fluid collection (Figures 2.15 and 2.16).

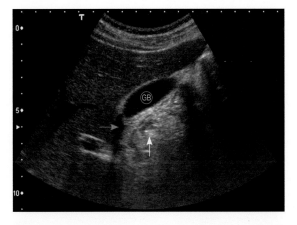

**Figure 2.15** Abdominal ultrasound demonstrating posterior enhancement (area of increased echogenicity (white arrow) behind the fluid-filled gallbladder (GB). Also note adjacent edge-shadowing artifact (blue arrow).

CHAPTER 2

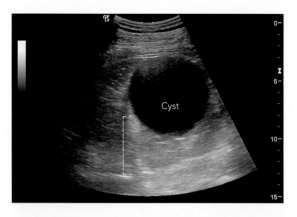

**Figure 2.16** Image of a large renal cyst. The high fluid content causes posterior enhancement deep to the structure (white bracket).

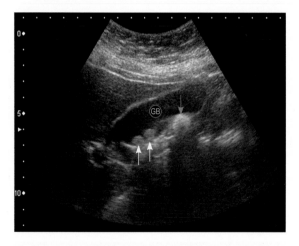

**Figure 2.17** Gallstone (blue arrow) inside the gallbladder (GB) demonstrating acoustic shadowing. Note that the smaller stones (white arrows) are not heavily calcified and cast a less dense shadow.

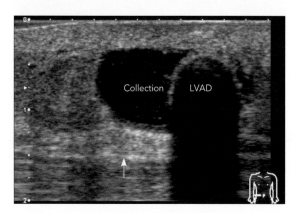

## Acoustic shadowing

Acoustic shadowing occurs due to either complete attenuation or reflection of the sound wave. In the presence of high-density tissues, e.g., bone, metal, and calcification, this is due to attenuation of the sound wave. This prevents further propagation and transmission of the wave and causes deeper tissue to produce fewer or no echoes, and therefore appear echo void. This gives the appearance of a casting shadow. Acoustic shadowing is typically seen behind ribs, gallstones, and calcified atheromatous plaque (Figure 2.17). The presence of an acoustic shadow will preclude the visualization of the underlying structures (Figure 2.18). This is particularly important if a pleural or mediastinal interventional procedure is to be performed and the acoustic shadow from the rib or sternum prevents adequate visualization of the biopsy needle along the biopsy track.

Acoustic shadowing, when caused by reflection, is generally seen at air or gas interfaces where 99% of the sound wave is reflected with little or no distal transmission and fewer echoes.

All shadows can be either clean or dirty. Clean shadows usually occur with large objects or, if small, objects with smooth surface, e.g., ribs and stones. Dirty shadows are seen with small objects with irregular surfaces or gaseous material, e.g., bowel gas (Figures 2.19a and b—clip) or air bronchograms (Figure 2.20).

## Contact artifact

This is caused when there is poor contact between the transducer and the skin surface. Using more gel or changing the angle of the transducer reduces this artifact (Figures 2.21a and b).

**Figure 2.18** Anterior chest wall ultrasound in a patient with a left ventricular assist device (LVAD). This shows acoustic shadowing mimicking a rib shadow and precludes visualization of any structures lying below. Note is also made of an adjacent echo-poor fluid collection, causing posterior enhancement (arrow).

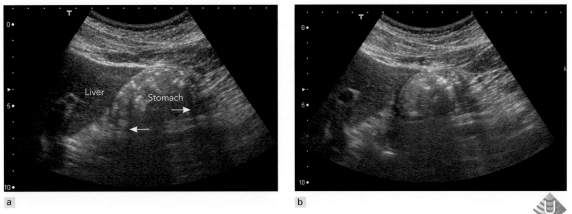

**Figure 2.19** Upper abdominal ultrasound performed in the epigastric region. (a) Echogenic air bubbles within the stomach cast "dirty shadows" (arrows). (b) Video showing echogenic air bubbles swirling within the stomach. View E-book for ultrasound clip or watch it at http://goo.gl/5ws3cG.

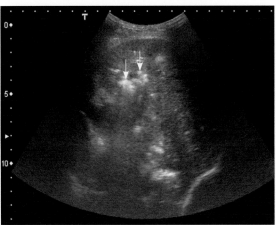

**Figure 2.20** Thoracic ultrasound demonstrating lobar consolidation, with bright echogenic air bronchograms (arrows) that cause "dirty" acoustic shadowing.

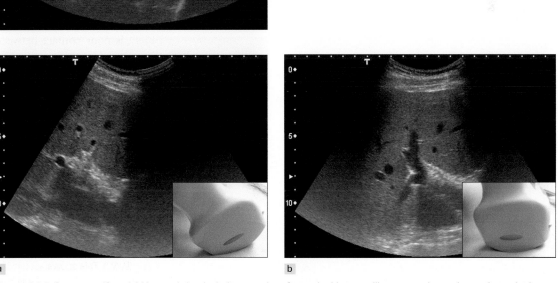

**Figure 2.21** Contact artifact. (a) Upper abdominal ultrasound performed with a curvilinear transducer shows that only the left side of the transducer is in direct contact with the skin. (b) By angling the artifact, the entire transducer face is now in contact with the skin.

CHAPTER 2

# ULTRASOUND CONTROLS— "KNOBOLOGY"

Thoracic ultrasound is performed using real-time gray-scale B- (brightness) mode scanning. Other imaging modes (A—amplitude and M—motion scanning) are not routinely used.

Most freestanding ultrasound machines have a large number of controls and functions (Figure 2.22). However, in everyday practice only a limited number of these controls are actually used for image optimization. The aim of this section is to provide a working knowledge of the ultrasound control panel and key controls that can be adjusted to optimize the ultrasound settings to ensure a good quality image.

When initially familiarizing yourself with ultrasound, a systematic approach to adjusting the controls can be helpful. Typically the key controls can be adjusted in the following order: depth, focus, time gain compensation, gain, and dynamic range.

## Depth

The depth control allows the location of the area of interest to be adjusted on the screen. Initially, in order to obtain an overview of the area to be scanned, a greater depth of view should be set than will be needed when the area of interest has been clearly identified. Once the area of interest has been identified, the depth of view should be reduced to allow its maximum visualization (Figure 2.23a—c).

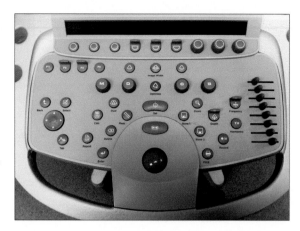

**Figure 2.22** Normal control panel on a Zonare ultrasound machine.

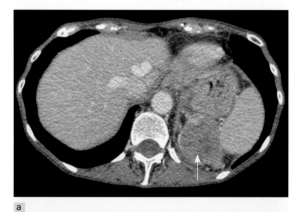

a

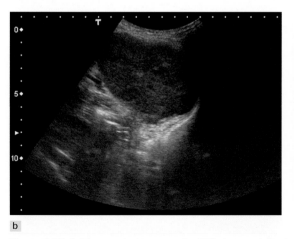

b

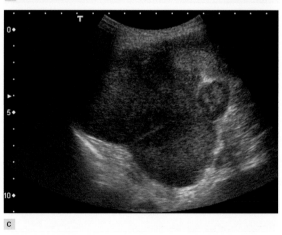

c

**Figure 2.23** Axial computed tomography (CT) shows a left adrenal metastasis (arrow). (a) On ultrasound the metastasis appears as a lobulated hypoechoic mass. (b) By decreasing the depth, the metastasis is now more appropriately sited in the center of the image.

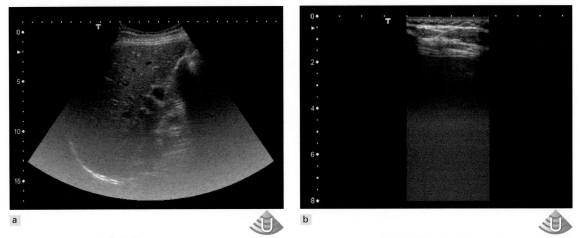

a                    b

**Figure 2.24** Focal zones. Upper abdominal ultrasound performed using a (a) curvilinear and (b) linear transducer. Both videos demonstrate how adjusting the focal zone can alter the image quality and resolution at a given depth. Location of the focal zone is indicated by the small white triangle adjacent to the measuring scale at the left of the screen. The triangle moves downward as the focal zone is moved deeper. View E-book for ultrasound clips or watch them at http://goo.gl/v9JnMq and http://goo.gl/i63Vjw.

## Focus

Focusing enables the ultrasound beam to be narrowed manually. This not only improves the lateral resolution (ability to separate two adjacent structures at a given depth), but also concentrates the intensity of the transmitted wave and echo signal over a desired depth (focal zone) that corresponds to the region of interest (Figure 2.24a and b—clips). Depending upon the size and depth of the region of interest, the operator can create single or multiple focal zones. Multiple focal zones will produce a long, narrow beam and improve the overall image quality; however, it will slow the pulse repetition frequency (number of sound waves emitted by the transducer per second) and frame rate, leading to a jerkier image.

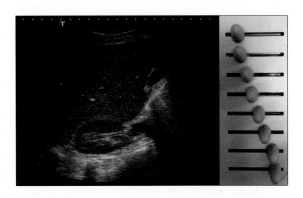

**Figure 2.25** Correct time gain compensation (TGC) setting.

## Time gain compensation (TGC)

Because ultrasound waves are attenuated as they pass through tissue, the signal returning to the transducer is less than that transmitted. As a result, the echoes from deeper structures are always much weaker than those from superficial structures. To produce an image and compensate for this, the returning sound signal requires some form of amplification. This is achieved by the TGC control, where the operator can control the degree of amplification at different positions in the ultrasound image. The near field usually requires no amplification, whereas the far field will require increasing amplification with increasing distance from the transducer. The overall aim is to produce an image of uniform brightness. On the ultrasound machine the default TGC setting is usually set diagonally (Figure 2.25). It is important to always check the TGC settings before scanning, as they may have been adjusted by the previous user (Figures 2.26 and 2.27).

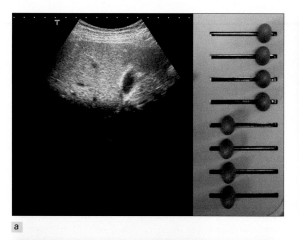

a

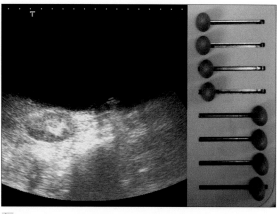

b

**Figure 2.26** Hepatic ultrasound showing incorrect TGC settings. (a) Increased near-field amplification and brightness, and decreased far-field amplification and echo loss. (b) Decreased near-field and increased far-field amplification. (c) Increased near and far amplification with decreased mid-field amplification.

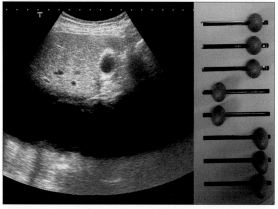

c

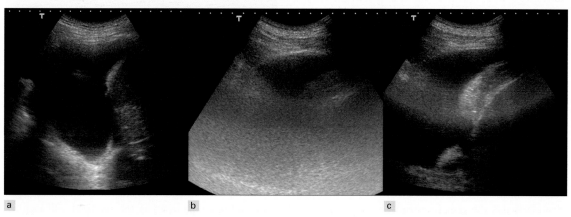

a                                  b                                  c

**Figure 2.27** Thoracic ultrasound showing a simple left pleural effusion with (a) correct TGC setting, (b) incorrect TGC setting with increased far-field brightness that forms a veil and hides the underlying effusion, and (c) incorrect TGC setting with increased mid-field brightness.

**Figure 2.28** (a) Contrast-enhanced CT demonstrates a left upper lobe bronchogenic carcinoma (arrow). (b) On ultrasound this is clearly identified as a hypoechoic mass with evidence of invasion through the pleura (P) into the chest wall (CW). (c) Reducing the overall gain darkens the image. (d) Increasing the gain brightens the image.

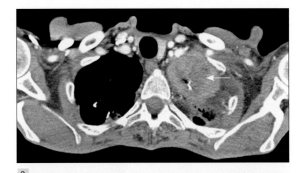

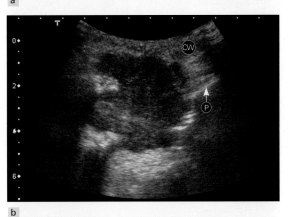

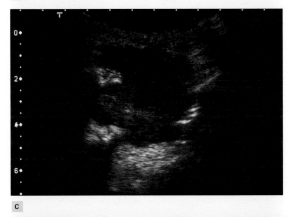

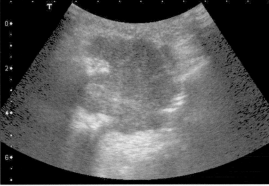

## Gain control

This affects the brightness of the entire image by amplifying the overall signal received. Increasing the gain enhances all the echoes uniformly and will brighten the image; however, it can cause loss of detail, making it more difficult to distinguish adjacent structures, and artifactually produce the appearance of echoes in areas of low echogenicity, such as fluid, potentially making anechoic effusions appear echogenic. Decreasing the gain will darken the image, causing structures to be lost (Figure 2.28a—d). Most beginners starting scanning have a tendency to set the gain too high.

## Dynamic range

This determines how many shades of gray or range of echoes are demonstrated on an image and the contrast resolution of the image. Altering the dynamic range allows subtle changes within tissues to be differentiated. If the image is degraded by low-level noise or artifacts, reducing the dynamic range can improve the overall image quality (Figure 2.29).

## Zoom

Magnifies the region of interest, but the image can appear "grainier" (Figure 2.30).

## Sector width

Varying the sector width alters the field of view and resolution of the ultrasound image. For practical purposes, when altering the sector width it is important to achieve a careful balance between good spatial resolution and a field of view that is not clipped too tightly, so that the relationship of the region of interest and surrounding structures may be assessed.

CHAPTER 2

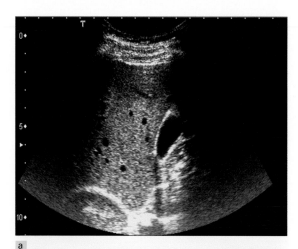

a

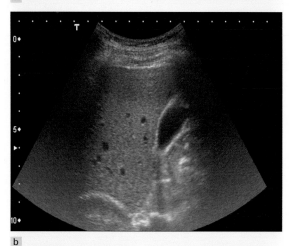

b

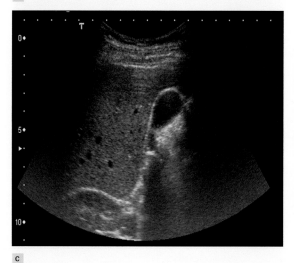

c

**Figure 2.29** Dynamic range control that is (a) set too low, (b) set too high, (c) optimal.

## Freeze

The freeze control captures the image displayed on the screen at that moment in time. Most ultrasound machines have a cine loop function whereby using the tracker ball, the operator can scroll back through the preceding several seconds of the scan, frame by frame. This allows a series of images to be reviewed and the most appropriate image stored.

## Calipers

Once an image has been captured and frozen on the screen, the caliper control allows the distance between two points to be measured.

## Optimize

All ultrasound machines now have an optimize control. This is a "get out of jail free" control that can be used if manual control adjustment doesn't improve the image quality adequately.

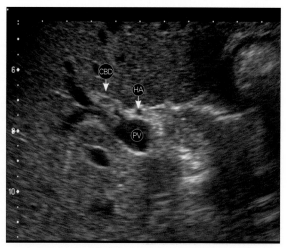

**Figure 2.30** Zooming allows the area of interest, which in this example represents the portal vein (PV), hepatic artery (HA), and common bile duct (CBD), to be magnified.

# DOPPLER IMAGING

When sound strikes a moving object a Doppler shift occurs. This is the change in the perceived frequency relative to the transmitted frequency. It is dependent on the angle, velocity, and direction of blood flow. If the sound wave is perpendicular to the moving object, no Doppler shift occurs.

## Color doppler

Doppler shift is usually depicted as shades of color. Traditionally, red represents blood flow moving toward the probe and blue away from the transducer (Figure 2.31—clip). It is important to remember that red does not represent an artery or blue a vein. If the Doppler flow signal is poor, a pulsed wave can be applied to a vessel, which provides an audible spectral trace that enables flow in arteries and veins to be differentiated and allows simple velocity measurements to be taken (Figures 2.32a and b—clip).

## Power doppler

Power Doppler mode permits the detection of low-velocity flow. It is more sensitive than color Doppler, as the returning echoes from the blood cells are analyzed by their power spectrum instead of by frequency shift. Power Doppler is used when small blood vessels need to be detected reliably, e.g., intercostal arteries, and when measurement of speed or direction of flow is not required (Figures 2.33a and b—clip).

**Figure 2.31** Carotid Doppler ultrasound shows flow within the common carotid artery and adjacent internal jugular vein. View E-book for ultrasound clip or watch it at http://goo.gl/G4wtPy.

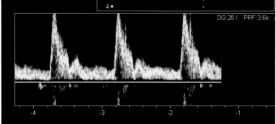

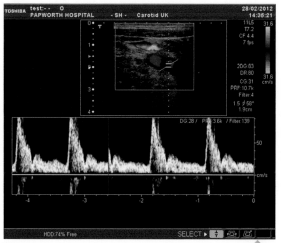

a    b

**Figure 2.32** (a) Pulsed-wave Doppler shows the typical spectral trace of an artery, which in this case corresponds to the internal carotid artery. (b) Ultrasound clip of (a). View E-book for ultrasound clip or watch it at http://goo.gl/gTNw9P.

CHAPTER 2

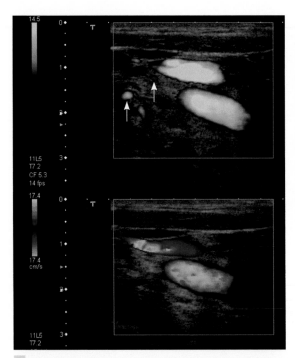

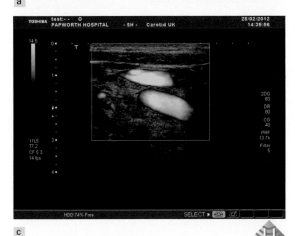

a

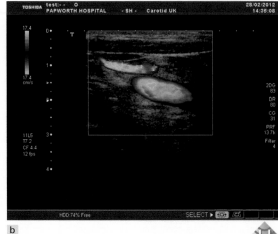

b

**Figure 2.33** (a) Power Doppler shows flow within smaller-caliber low-velocity vessels (arrows) that was not evident on the color Doppler image (lower image). (b) Color Doppler. (c) Power Doppler. View E-book for ultrasound clips or watch them at http://goo.gl/JdVyKH and http://goo.gl/qRUjJn.

c

## TIPS FOR CLINICAL PRACTICE

- Spend time optimizing the image.
- Always adjust the ultrasound controls in a systematic order as described.
- When scanning, ensure the focal zone corresponds to the region of interest.
- In larger patients always use a curvilinear transducer, as a linear transducer will never provide adequate depth penetration even for superficial structures.
- If all else fails, use more ultrasound gel.

Of all imaging modalities, ultrasound is probably the most operator- and patient body habitus-dependent. The ultrasound controls will therefore always require different degrees of adjusting to achieve a diagnostic quality image. Generally, the optimal ultrasound settings are a matter of personal preference based on practical experience and expertise.

## REFERENCES

1. TS Curry, JE Dowdy, RC Murry. Christensen's physics of diagnostic radiology. *Ultrasound* 1990; 20:323–371.

2. RF Farr, PJ Allisy-Roberts. Physics for medical imaging. *Imaging with Ultrasound* 1997; 7:183–212.

3. MK Feldman, S Katyal, MS Blackwood. Continuing medical education: US artifacts. *Radiographics* 2009; 29(4):1179–1189.

4. MA Sandler, BL Madrazo, R Walter, *et al.* Ultrasound case of the day. Duplication artifact (mirror image artifact). *Radiographics* 1987; 7(5):1025–8.

CHAPTER 2

## MCQ 1

 Which of the following statements are correct (multiple answers possible)?

Higher-frequency transducers have:

**a.** No need for gel coupling.

**b.** Good depth penetration.

**c.** Higher attenuation in tissue.

**d.** Improved resolution in the near field.

**e.** Large diameters.

## MCQ 2

 What artifacts are demonstrated in this image (multiple answers possible)?

**a.** Edge artifact.

**b.** Posterior enhancement.

**c.** Contact artifact.

**d.** Reverberation.

**e.** Side lobe artifact.

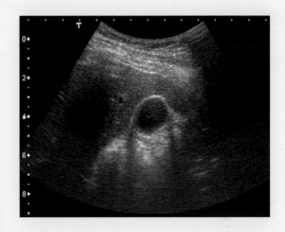

## MCQ 3

 Which controls need to be adjusted to improve this image (multiple answers possible)?

**a.** Focal zone.

**b.** Depth.

**c.** TGC.

**d.** Zoom.

**e.** Transducer–patient contact.

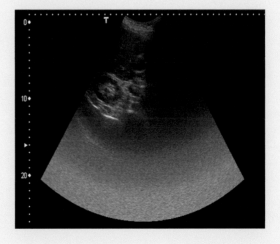

CHAPTER 2

## MCQ 4

**Q** Which controls need to be adjusted to optimize this image of the liver?

a. Focal zone.
b. Dynamic range.
c. Sector width.
d. TGC.
e. Depth.

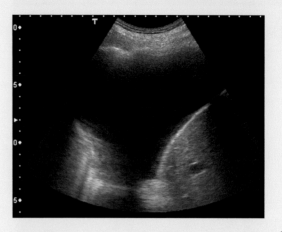

## ANSWERS

**1.** c, d

See Chapter 2 for more detail.

**2.** a, b, c

See labeled image (right) illustrating the relevant artifacts and Chapter 2 for further explanation: a = edge artifact, b = posterior enhancement; c = contact artifact.

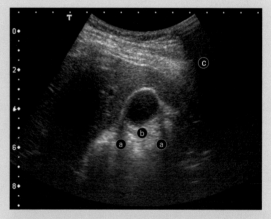

**3.** a, b, e

See labeled image (right) for illustration. This image is set too deep (b). A depth of 12–15 cm would allow optimum visualization of the structures. The focal zone (a)—white triangle adjacent to the measurement scale—is also set too deep. There is loss of transducer–skin contact on the right of the image (e).

**4.** d

There is not uniform brightness across the image. The TGC controls are not in alignment (see Chapter 2).

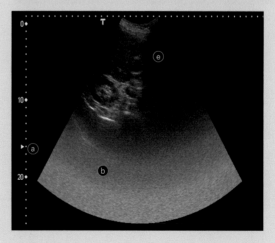

# Getting Started: Bringing the Ultrasound Machine to the Patient

Luke Garske, John Coucher, and Scott King

## BEDSIDE ULTRASOUND: INTRODUCTION

*Scenario 1:* Dr. Smith is asked to review Mr. A. in his clinic. The chest x-ray (CXR) shows blunting of the right costophrenic angle, suggesting the presence of a moderate-sized pleural effusion. Clinical examination findings are equivocal. He prepares and repositions the patient on the examination couch. An ultrasound examination of the right hemithorax reveals no pleural fluid, suggesting that the CXR appearance is due to pleural thickening. Appropriate further investigation is immediately arranged.

*Scenario 2:* Dr. Jones is called to the intensive care unit at 2 a.m. to review a ventilated patient whose gas exchange is deteriorating rapidly. The CXR reveals a left pleural effusion, and there are no other clinically identifiable reversible factors. However, the patient is obese and has multiple limb fractures, increasing the difficulty of chest drainage. Nursing staff position the patient for a left chest ultrasound, while Dr. Jones prepares the ultrasound machine. Ultrasound reveals a deep, accessible effusion with no loculation. She places a mark on the patient's skin, with appropriate distances measured with ultrasound, so that she can immediately insert a chest tube with minimal risk of complications.

Ultrasound can be helpful in a wide range of differing clinical environments. Each environment presents unique technical challenges to the successful acquisition of an optimal image of thoracic anatomy and pleural pathology. This chapter will summarize common principles and practical suggestions that will guide you to achieve optimal ultrasound imaging and interpretation in whatever clinical scenario you are presented with.

## PREPARATION

A useful and successful ultrasound examination depends on the optimal preparation, arrangement, use, and interaction of the key components (Video 3.1), namely:

- Patient.
- Ultrasound machine and associated equipment.
- Operator.
- Scanning environment and ergonomics.

These components should be reviewed prior to each examination. However, this process will vary, depending on whether the procedure is elective or emergent, where the procedure is being done (clinic, bedside, or operating theater), and whether the procedure is purely diagnostic or to guide intervention.

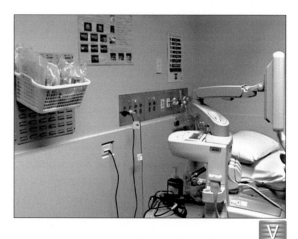

**Video 3.1** Demonstration of the steps involved in preparing to perform a pleural ultrasound examination. View E-book for video clip or watch it at http://goo.gl/NTK8PX.

3

## Patient factors

Optimal positioning of the patient is essential for successful pleural ultrasound. This is because pleural effusions are mobile and tend to move to the most dependent part of the pleural space. In a patient who is ambulatory, positioning the patient erect will generally give the best diagnostic results. In this position, fluid will preferentially accumulate in the posterior costophrenic recesses, where it can be readily seen from a posterior approach. Additionally, the liver and spleen can be easily identified, serving as landmarks. The easiest way to achieve this position is to sit the patient on the edge of a bed or on a stool, leaning slightly forward, with a pillow on their lap. Alternatively, they may sit on an adjustable rotating chair, leaning forward against the back of the chair (Figure 3.1). The scapulae are moved forward so they do not obstruct the ultrasound examination. This is often the optimal patient position for diagnostic ultrasound (Scenario 1).

However, a variety of patient positions may be successfully used.[1] An optimal position maximizes the chances of a successful and time-efficient examination, and considers patient comfort and stability. If an intervention is planned, optimal positioning also considers procedural access. Sometimes, several different degrees of obliquity of patient position need to be tried to facilitate movement of pleural fluid, so there is a sufficient depth of fluid at the site requiring procedural access.

With a less mobile or unconscious patient, a different approach has to be adopted. When the patient is supine, fluid will preferentially accumulate posteriorly, where the probe cannot be placed. Therefore, the patient needs to be rolled toward the lateral decubitus position (Figure 3.2), and propped up posteriorly with pillows or patient positioning pads (Figure 3.3). In this position, fluid in the uppermost hemithorax will preferentially accumulate medially adjacent to the spine, but larger effusions usually also extend superiorly from the lateral costophrenic recess, as well as anteriorly. The ultrasound probe can readily access the lateral and posterolateral aspects of the uppermost hemithorax to guide intervention (Scenario 2).

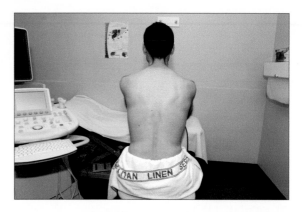

**Figure 3.1** Patient is positioned for erect scanning, seated on a stool, leaning forward over a chair back or pillow.

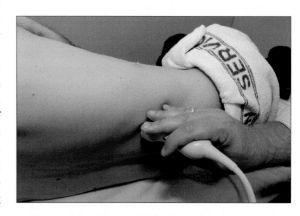

**Figure 3.2** Patient being scanned in the lateral decubitus position, with the effusion side up.

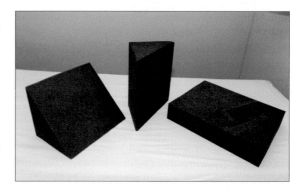

**Figure 3.3** Selection of foam patient positioning pads for comfortable support and immobilization. These are covered when in use to keep them clean.

If the patient is immobile, or the target does not move when the patient changes position (for example, a loculated effusion or a pleural-based lesion), other positions can be tried until a satisfactory view is obtained. Positioning should consider the expected location of the target beneath the chest wall, and should avoid structures such as the scapula that will obstruct the ultrasound beam. Small changes in position and posture can radically improve sonographic visualization.

It is important to ensure that enough patient clothing is removed prior to chest ultrasound, especially bra straps. Clothing can prevent adequate probe travel, and ultrasound gel tends to leave salty marks, which don't wash out easily. Covering the patient's waistline with a towel is also recommended to protect clothing from gel.

## Ultrasound machine and probes

- Ensure you have access to an adequate power supply, and that the electrical needs of the ultrasound machine will not exceed local capacity (especially relevant in environments with multiple electrical equipment such as intensive care).
- Most machines take a significant amount of time to start up. Turn the machine on as soon as possible to minimize the effect of this enforced delay.
- Ensure you have the correct ultrasound probe available, connected, and selected (Figure 3.4). In patients with pleural effusion, the best images are generally obtained with a low-frequency probe (typically 3–5 MHz), which penetrates more deeply, whereas higher-resolution images of the chest wall or pleural layers are generally obtained with a high-frequency probe (typically 8–12 MHz).
- Ensure you clean the probe before use.
- Enter the patient's details into the ultrasound machine so that these will be recorded with the image.

### TIPS FOR CLINICAL PRACTICE

After preparing the machine and probe, tap or touch the probe surface with a finger to ensure the correct probe is selected and working (see Video 3.1). If no movement is seen on the screen, check that any screen freeze/hold function is off, and that the 2D gain is adequately turned up. Applying gel to the active probe face should also make the screen image brighter.

- Select the correct preset on machines that have this feature. Advanced machines have multiple presets that affect the way the image is processed by the machine. The abdominal preset is usually optimal for pleural ultrasound. Using the wrong one, e.g., "musculoskeletal," can degrade the image or make normal appearances look abnormal.
- Check that the TGC is initially set equal across all depths of examination, the focal zone is at approximately the correct depth for the examination, and the 2D gain is turned up.

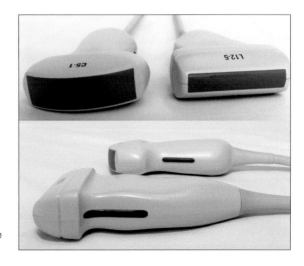

**Figure 3.4** Ultrasound probes. Upper left: Curvilinear C5-1 probe uses frequencies 1–5 MHz and is good for scanning effusions. Upper right: Linear L12-5 probe uses frequencies 5–12 MHz and is better for superficial structures, including the chest wall. Lower: Note the probe markers visible on the probe sides.

CHAPTER 3

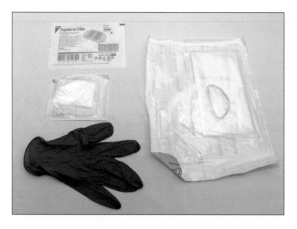

**Figure 3.5** A variety of materials can be used to cover the probe.

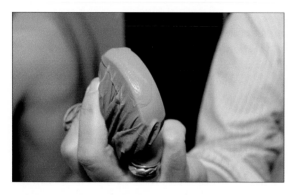

**Figure 3.6** A glove with gel inside can be used to protect the probe while scanning in contaminated environments.

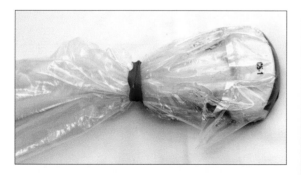

**Figure 3.7** Sterile probe and cord cover with gel inside, which is used to scan in sterile environments.

**Figure 3.8** Tegaderm dressing on probe (with gel underneath) used to protect the probe face from blood or body fluids while scanning.

## Operator

Review of the patient's most recent CXR or computed tomography (CT) scan is mandatory immediately prior to scanning and intervention. When integrated with clinical information, this will ensure the aim of the procedure is clear. This is particularly important if focal pleural lesions or loculated collections are suspected, so the examination can be tailored. Review of recent imaging also prevents any possible errors (for example, scanning the wrong side if patients have bilateral effusions). The identification of a pneumothorax or hydropneumothorax on a recent CXR/CT may enable more efficient interpretation of thoracic ultrasound by less expert sonographers.

## Scanning environment and ergonomics

- Appropriate background lighting optimizes viewing conditions for the screen and avoids glare. Where possible, use dimmable lighting with window blinds and curtains to exclude natural light.
- Required equipment includes gel, towels, and tissue paper, and equipment to clean the machine and probes.
- Appropriate probe covers will be required if working in a contaminated environment or for intervention (Figures 3.5–3.8).

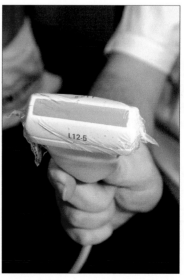

- If planning to mark a site for drainage, an indelible marker pen is less likely to wash off with antiseptic.
- A web view workstation, picture archiving and communication system (PACS) workstation, or even film viewing box close to the scanner is helpful to assist in correlation of radiology, as well as comparison of previous ultrasound scans.
- The gel bottle should be within easy reach.
- A probe holder should be within easy reach to secure the probe when not in use.

We have discussed positioning the patient, operator, and machine, but to efficiently and effectively perform pleural ultrasound we need to consider the interaction of all three elements, and adjust to differing clinical scenarios. In general, the patient, machine, and operator should be in an equilateral triangular arrangement, so that the operator has comfortable equal access to the patient and the machine. The exact positioning required to achieve this will depend on which hand the probe is held in and which part of the thorax is examined (Video 3.1, Figures 3.9–3.14). If you are performing real-time ultrasound-guided pleural intervention, it is preferable

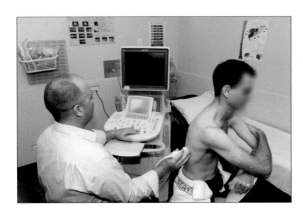

**Figure 3.9** Ergonomic positioning: right-handed operator scanning right hemithorax. Patient on stool.

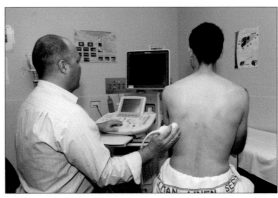

**Figure 3.10** Ergonomic positioning. Right-handed operator scanning left hemithorax. Patient on stool.

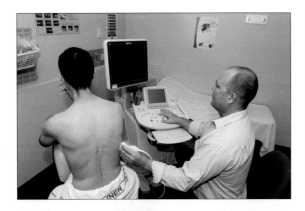

**Figure 3.11** Ergonomic positioning. Left-handed operator scanning right hemithorax. Patient on stool.

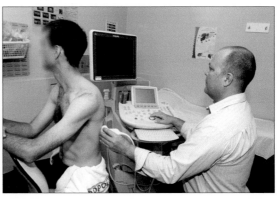

**Figure 3.12** Ergonomic positioning. Left-handed operator scanning left hemithorax. Patient on stool.

CHAPTER 3

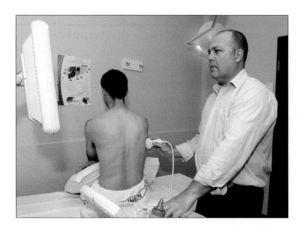

**Figure 3.13** Ergonomic positioning. Operator standing with screen raised. Patient seated on raised bed.

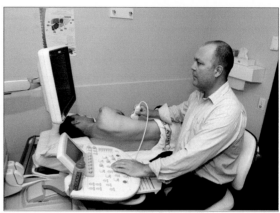

**Figure 3.14** Ergonomic positioning: lateral decubitus. Operator rests the arm holding the probe on the patient's hip.

| Table 3.1 **Ergonomics to minimize injury to the operator** |
| --- |
| Keep head above spine, don't lean forward |
| Ultrasound monitor close to eye level |
| Upper arm close to body |
| Patient region to be scanned at optimal height for the operator |
| If doing prolonged scanning, vary between sitting and standing |
| Ensure the operator is comfortable while scanning, with no strain |
| *Source*: Furlow B, *Radiol Technol* 2002;74:137–50; quiz 152–3, 135–6. |

to have the monitor in line with the operative field, to allow ease of viewing of the ultrasound image and the procedural site. A series of suggested principles of positioning (Table 3.1) may minimize the risk of repetitive strain injury to the operator.[2] A height-adjustable chair for the patient or operator is invaluable.

## PERFORMING THE SCAN

### Probe manipulation

Correct manual control of the probe helps to efficiently achieve an optimal image, while maintaining patient comfort (Video 3.2, Figures 3.15 and 3.16). Experienced operators hold the probe in various ways. We suggest the following guides to assist you to hold the probe so that firm pressure can be comfortably applied in a controlled manner, but probe angle and position can be easily and precisely adjusted:

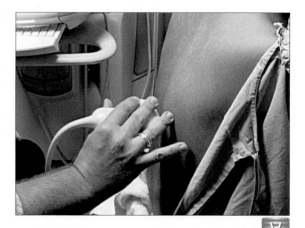

**Video 3.2** Video demonstration of correct probe manipulation and orientation. View E-book for video clip or watch it at http://goo.gl/zNJHtE.

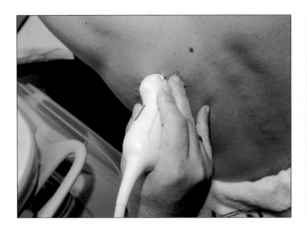
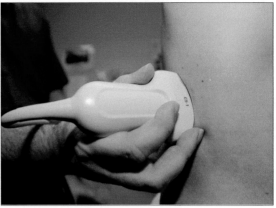

**Figures 3.15 and 3.16** Correct holding of the probe. The thumb and index finger are as close to the probe face as possible, with the little finger maintaining tactile contact with the patient. Other fingers wrap around the probe to support and stabilize.

- Hold the probe like a pencil, *not* like a knife or a piece of chalk, with fingers as low down the probe toward the transducer face as possible. This places the thumb and index finger as close to the transducer face as possible, where they can exert precise control. Don't be scared to get gel on your hands.
- Keep anchoring contact between the operator's probe hand and the patient's chest wall (e.g., with little finger). This gives a tactile sense of the probe's position and movement on the patient while the operator is looking at the image screen.
- Your thumb and index finger together are the key controllers of the probe. The remaining fingers exert some added control and are particularly useful for spreading pressure across the hand. This improves comfort if you are scanning for a prolonged time.
- If your fingers are long enough, try to curl them around the probe body.
- Avoid marked wrist angulation; the muscles moving the wrist are less precise in controlling the probe than the fingers.

### TIPS FOR CLINICAL PRACTICE

- Be generous with the gel. It is best and easier to place gel on the probe rather than the patient.
- Plenty of ultrasound gel ensures better exclusion of air from the transducer-gel-tissue interface since even minute amounts of air between the probe and patient's skin can degrade the ultrasound image. Frequent reapplications during the examination may be required. Dressings and even extensive body hair can prevent good coupling with the ultrasound transducer and may have to be removed to ensure a technically adequate examination.
- Before scanning the thorax, start scanning the left or right lateral/posterolateral upper abdominal wall. The liver, kidneys, or spleen need to be located anyway, and provide good targets to optimize the various machine settings before moving onto the thorax (see Video 3.2).

CHAPTER 3

## Probe orientation

Ultrasound requires examination of the region of interest in more than one plane, as this assists in identifying anatomic structures and artifacts, and assessing the margin for safety when guiding drainage. Usually for pleural ultrasound the region of interest will be examined in at least:

- A vertical/longitudinal plane, e.g., parasagittal plane for the anterior and posterior thorax, and coronal plane for the lateral thorax.
- An axial/transverse plane, or an oblique (between vertical and axial) plane. It may be preferable to examine with the probe aligned along the line of the intercostal space. This avoids acoustic shadowing from the ribs and allows a maximal acoustic window to the pleural space.

Recording and viewing images in a conventional orientation allows easier understanding and comparison of the images by yourself and others. The general convention for ultrasound is that the side of the probe with the marker should be displayed on the left side of the image screen, where there is a corresponding screen marker. The ultrasound probe marker is generally a notch, stripe, or light on the probe housing.

When the probe is orientated with the ultrasound beam in a predominantly vertical/longitudinal plane, the convention is to place the probe marker toward the head of the patient.[3] In a vertical plane, anatomically superior structures will therefore be on the left side of the screen, with inferiorly placed structures on the right of the screen (Video 3.2, Figures 3.17a and b). When the probe is oriented with the ultrasound beam in a predominantly axial/transverse plane, the convention is to place the probe marker toward the left side of the operator's view of the patient (Video 3.2, Figures 3.18a and b, and 3.19). This corresponds to viewing the structures within the ultrasound beam from the direction of the patient's feet.[3] For axial images, the anatomic orientation will vary depending on the part of the thorax being examined, with the left side of the screen image generally corresponding to:

- Anatomic left for the posterior thorax.
- Anatomic anterior for the left lateral thorax.
- Anatomic right for the anterior thorax.
- Anatomic posterior for the right lateral thorax.

When examining the thorax, the probe is frequently obliquely aligned along the intercostal space. In an oblique plane, the probe is often held in a plane that is slightly more vertical than transverse, to maintain awareness of the position of the hemidiaphragm and subphrenic structures (Video 3.2, Figures 3.20a and b). Thus, in an oblique plane the probe marker is often toward the patient's head.[3]

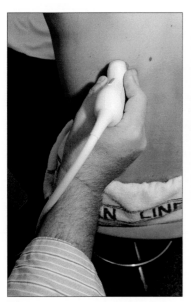

a

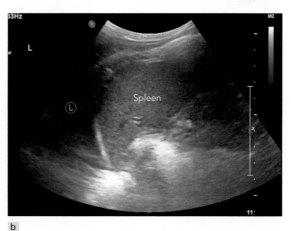

b

**Figure 3.17** (a) Conventional orientation of the probe in a vertical/longitudinal plane on the patient's left, with probe marker toward the patient's head. (b) Corresponding ultrasound image: aerated lung (L) to the left of screen (superiorly) and spleen centrally and toward the right (inferiorly).

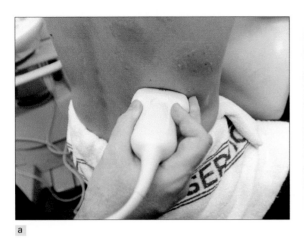

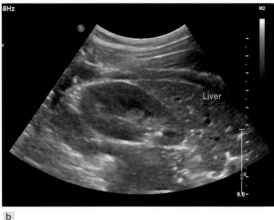

**Figure 3.18** (a) Conventional orientation of the probe in an axial/transverse plane, examining the right posterior aspect of the patient with the probe marker toward the operator's left (and the patient's anatomic left side). (b) The corresponding ultrasound image shows the right kidney to the left of the screen, with the liver to the right of the screen.

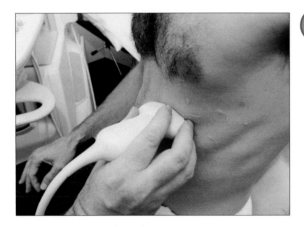

**Figure 3.19** Conventional orientation of the probe in an axial plane, anterior thorax. The probe marker is toward the operator's left (and the patient's anatomic right side).

## TIPS FOR CLINICAL PRACTICE

You can check which side of the probe corresponds to the marker by:

- Confirming that the direction of probe movement corresponds to the correct direction of movement of the tissues on the screen.

- Applying ultrasound gel initially on one end of the transducer while looking at the screen image (also confirms the image is not frozen).

- Tapping one end of the transducer with your finger, and confirming that the end being tapped corresponds to the expected side of the screen image.

CHAPTER 3

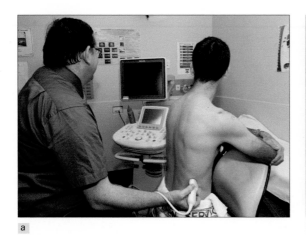
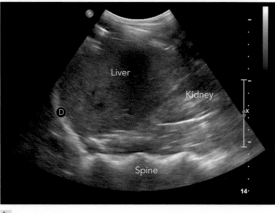

**Figure 3.20** (a) Conventional orientation of the probe in an oblique plane (to allow scanning in the intercostal space) on the patient's right side. The probe marker is toward the patient's head. (b) The corresponding ultrasound image shows the hemidiaphragm (D) on the left side of the image (superior), the liver centrally, and the right kidney to the right side of the image (inferiorly). The spine is responsible for the undulating echogenic line on the inferior part of the image (medial to the liver).

Following this convention helps ensure that the operator has correct spatial awareness at all times and can correctly localize all structures. However, this rigid convention needs to be balanced with a flexible examination technique. Frequently adjusting the direction and position of the probe allows the best quality images to be acquired while building up a three-dimensional appreciation of the abnormality. While we advocate this orientation convention, we also emphasize the freehand, interactive, and unconstrained nature of ultrasound compared to other imaging modalities.

## RECORDING RESULTS: ARCHIVING ULTRASOUND IMAGES

It is essential to make a record of your findings. Storing the images from any diagnostic ultrasound procedure is advisable, as this provides:

- A medicolegal record.
- Documentation of change over time.
- Potential for a second opinion from medical colleagues.
- Teaching material.

Most modern ultrasound machines are Digital Imaging and Communications in Medicine (DICOM) compatible. This means that recorded images can be readily stored and displayed on a PACS or using a DICOM server. DICOM is a standard for digital medical images in much the same way that mp3 is for digital music files. PACSs are most commonly found in medical imaging departments and are advantageous for large-scale image storage and retrieval. Connecting a system to a PACS by cable or wirelessly can enable (1) review of previously stored images, (2) coregistration of a pre-existing CT chest data set to enable hybrid US-CT 3D navigation for intervention, and (3) patient work list functionality. A work list enables the operator to select the patient's name and other details directly from a list preentered by booking staff rather than having to enter them manually.

If you don't have access to a PACS, or if the administrative support required to manage a PACS is excessive for the volume of images requiring storage, a local method of image storage is required. Depending on the machine, the images can be stored on various forms of digital media, e.g., hard drive, CD, flash drive, or memory card, recorded onto video tape or DVD, or printed onto paper or film. If your ultrasound machine has a hard drive, consider a schedule for regular download of images from the machine for long-term storage on other media.

## POST-SCAN

### Etiquette and probe care

Ultrasound probes are delicate and expensive. The crystals within the transducer are easily damaged if dropped. They also carry some risks of transmitting infection between patients, and standard clinical hygiene measures and cleanliness should be applied. The probe transducer face may be damaged by alcohol-based solutions such as antiseptic, so contact with these should be avoided (follow manufacturer's instructions). Where there is any potential for contamination with blood or other bodily secretions, the probe should be protected from these with a disposable cover. After completing an examination, the probe should be cleaned with gentle wiping, followed by the use of a compatible cleaning spray for infection control (Table 3.2).

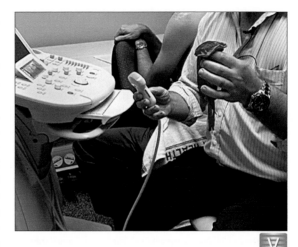

**Video 3.3** Demonstration of different methods of probe protection. View E-book for video clip or watch it at http://goo.gl/3ZU7P0.

---

**Table 3.2 Suggested etiquette at the end of an ultrasound examination**

1. Ensure the probe is secured in machine holder (where provided) and safe from accidental damage to the transducer face. Leave probe and electrical cables untangled and clear of machine wheels. Probe cable covers can be stripped off if left near wheels.

2. Ensure all gel is removed, and the probe is clean (including spray to the probe grooves).

3. Leave equipment, e.g., keyboard and screen, clean and ready to use.

4. If the machine is to be used again soon, it is routine to leave it powered up, but ideally the screen should be turned off when not in use for prolonged periods. Older ultrasound scanners may "burn" a static image into the screen if left powered up for prolonged periods.

## GUIDING INTERVENTION

Ultrasound can be used to guide chest intervention in two distinct modes, as detailed in the following sections.

### Real-time ultrasound guidance

Real-time ultrasound guidance provides accurate control of needle insertion with continuous ultrasound imaging. This provides minimal risk of unintended organ puncture, and precise administration of local anesthesia. This is an advantage when the target is small and there are sensitive structures nearby to be avoided. However, these procedures require a high degree of manual dexterity to keep the needle and probe face aligned appropriately.

CHAPTER 3

The same preliminary steps described previously are used. The patient must be in a comfortable stable position with adequate access for the interventional equipment. The machine settings must be carefully optimized before the procedure to obtain the clearest possible view. This is important, as the probe cover tends to degrade the image, and the room lighting level cannot be dimmed as much to optimize the screen view. Mark the site of the target and the optimum probe position/direction, before cleaning the skin with antiseptic; this facilitates the application of the drape fenestration in the correct position and orientation. The sterile drape requires a generous fenestration to allow adequate access for the probe and interventional equipment. Sterile transparent drapes are available to cover the controls of the ultrasound machine to allow the controls to be manipulated by the operator during the procedure. Sterile gel is commonly used to exclude air from between the transducer face and patient while maintaining sterility of the operating field. Sterile covers over the ultrasound probe are generally used, with the use of gel within the sterile sleeve, and an elastic band or tie to ensure the sleeve remains tightly around the transducer face, with no air pockets. It is often helpful to rest part of the hand holding the probe on the patient's skin to prevent it moving during the procedure. A generous amount of lignocaine should be used in the superficial skin, as the probe may move slightly and the exact site of needle insertion may be slightly different from the marked site. Care must be taken to minimize the amount of gel reaching the sampling needle when performing fine-needle aspiration of tissue, since the gel can prevent adequate cytology samples. When performing real-time guided procedures, it is critical to keep the needle and ultrasound probe appropiately aligned as the needle is inserted and advanced. The flatter the angle of needle insertion relative to the skin surface, the greater the beam reflection from the side of the needle, which makes the needle easier to see. It is often preferable to ensure the needle is visible along its entire length during insertion. With the in-plane technique, it is also important to identify the needle/cannula early after insertion into the skin, and then watch its movement when it is advanced; movement is more easily seen than a static needle (see Chapter 9).

## Ultrasound markup

The use of ultrasound to mark the position and depth of larger targets, particularly pleural effusions, offers a simpler and easier approach. However, the path the needle takes during pleural drainage may be significantly different from that hoped for during previous diagnostic ultrasound imaging, with a risk of inadvertent organ puncture. We suggest a series of steps to minimize this risk, which allow most pleural effusions of clinical significance to be successfully drained with this method (Video 3.4). Small effusions only accessible in one intercostal space, or with less than 1 cm depth as a safety margin, require real-time drainage. However, pleural effusions that are too small to be safely drained with ultrasound markup often do not require diagnostic sampling, so this is not a common scenario.

1.  Patient positioning. Ensure the patient is in the same position when you perform the ultrasound and the subsequent drainage procedure. Any change in position may cause fluid to shift internally, but also may cause the skin mark to move relative to deeper chest wall structures.

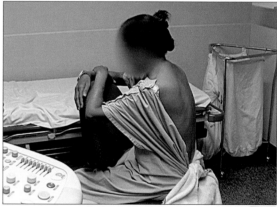

**Video 3.4** Video demonstrating a series of tips for ultrasound mark-up for drainage. View E-book for video clip or watch it at http://goo.gl/wPKffV.

**TIPS FOR CLINICAL PRACTICE**

A reversed needle can be used to indent the skin with a mark while gel is in place. After removing the gel you can then mark your selected insertion point with an indelible pen.

2. Select and mark the insertion site. Select a site with an adequate depth of effusion for the procedure planned. For example, for Seldinger chest tube insertion, allow at least 1–2 cm depth of fluid between entry of the needle into the pleural space and puncture of the lung. This will enable safe insertion of dilators with a tapered tip of 1 cm, which must fully enter the pleural space. Check that there is no intervening lung with the planned needle trajectory in all phases of deeper respiration, and that there is no risk of puncture of adjacent organs, such as the heart, liver, and spleen.[4] You will not be able to mark the site with a pen while gel is on the skin.

   It may be helpful to check the safety of depth of fluid in adjacent interspaces, to evaluate the risk in case your needle does not pass through the selected intercostal space.

3. Recheck the safety of drainage over the marked site in two planes. Recheck the depth of fluid remains adequate in two planes in all phases of respiration. One plane must be vertical to ensure your marked site will be above the diaphragm. Double-check the angle of the probe will correspond to your angle of needle insertion; it is most reproducible to keep the long axis of the probe perpendicular to the marked site, and subsequently insert the needle at the same angle.

**TIPS FOR CLINICAL PRACTICE**

Place the probe in the vertical/longitudinal plane on the skin mark (i.e., perpendicular to the skin), without looking at the screened image until the probe is held securely over the mark. Then check the screen image shows a safe needle path down the center of the screen.

You can measure the depth from skin puncture to entry of the needle into fluid. This is more accurate if you freeze the image with the least amount of probe pressure still able to maintain an image. However, the subsequent depth from skin to successful fluid aspiration can be greater than this due to (a) local anesthetic distending the tissues, and (b) stretching of the pleura with needle entry.

4. Clean off gel residue, and ensure you don't lose your mark with antiseptic. After removing gel again, it is prudent to remark the site to prevent it washing off with antiseptic solution. You can remove gel residue (which might harbor bacteria) with warm soapy water, prior to cleaning the skin with antiseptic. Ensure the needle enters the pleural space at the same perpendicular angle.

## CONCLUSION

We have summarized the practical knowledge and skills required to bring the ultrasound machine to the patient for both diagnostic and interventional scenarios. We have suggested a checklist for each of the key elements of the patient, machine, operator, and environment. The successful interaction of these elements requires planning and consideration of ergonomics, to ensure the comfort of the patient and the operator. We recommend holding the probe as close to the transducer face as possible. Image display should follow general ultrasound convention, with the probe marker oriented to the left of the screen image. With the probe in a vertical/longitudinal plane, the marker should be to the head of the patient, and when the probe is in an axial/transverse plane, the marker should be to the left side of the operator's view of the patient. The majority of pleural effusions can be successfully drained by ultrasound markup, but a series of steps are required to prevent the needle deviating substantially from the intended trajectory. Efficient and safe use of thoracic ultrasound is an acquired skill, which requires repeated practice in a range of clinical scenarios.

# REFERENCES

1. Diacon AH, Theron J, Bolliger CT. Transthoracic ultrasound for the pulmonologist. *Curr Opin Pulm Med* 2005; 11:307–12.

2. Furlow B. Ergonomics in the health care environment. *Radiol Technol* 2002; 74:137–50; quiz 152-3, 135–6.

3. McDicken W. *Diagnostic ultrasonics. Principles and use of instruments.* 3rd ed. Edinburgh: Churchill Livingstone, 1991:163.

4. Havelock T, Teoh R, Laws D, Gleeson F. Pleural procedures and thoracic ultrasound: British Thoracic Society Pleural Disease Guideline 2010. *Thorax* 2010; 65 (Suppl 2):ii61–76.

## MCQ 1

**Q** Which of the following four pictures demonstrate good ergonomics (positioning of the patient, machine, and operator in a way that ensures efficiency of examination and minimizes the risk of repetitive strain injury for the operator)? More than one response is possible.

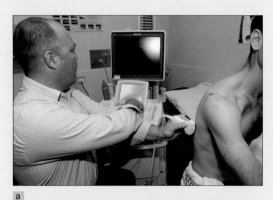

a

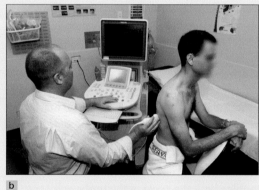

b

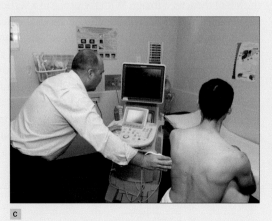

c

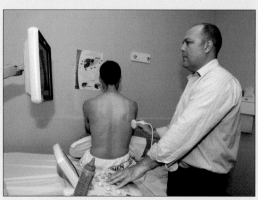

d

CHAPTER 3

## MCQ 2

**Q** Which of the following four pictures
demonstrate a good way to hold the probe?
More than one response is possible.

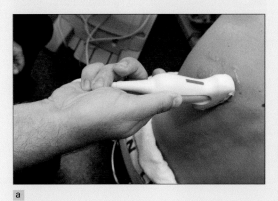

a

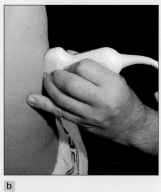

b

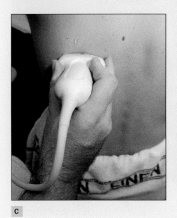

c

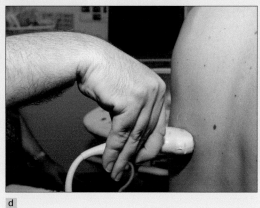

d

## MCQ 3

Q With the probe in the position shown (Figure a) and in the conventional orientation, which one of the following (Figures b–e) is the corresponding correct ultrasound image?

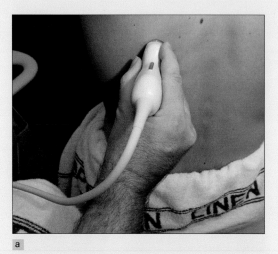

a

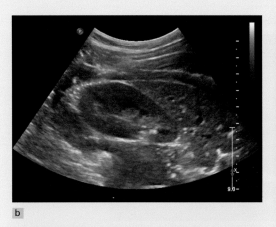

b

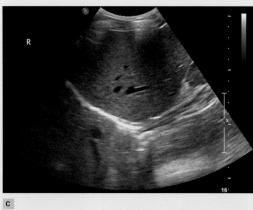

c

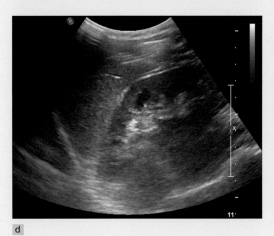

d

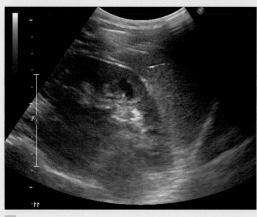

e

## MCQ 4

**Q** For the positions marked x and y on the blank ultrasound image (right):

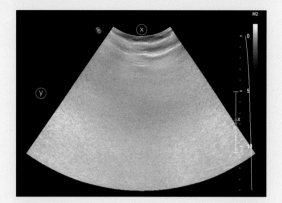

**a.** With the probe in the position shown.

   i.  Position 'x' on the ultrasound display is toward which part of the patient?

      – Anterior
      – Posterior
      – Superior
      – Inferior

   ii.  Position 'y' on the ultrasound display is toward which part of the patient?

      – Anterior
      – Posterior
      – Superior
      – Inferior

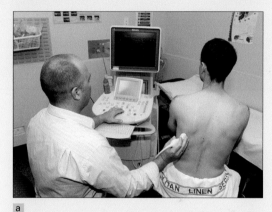

a

**b.** With the probe in the position shown.

   i.  Position 'x' on the ultrasound display is toward which part of the patient?

      – Left
      – Right
      – Anterior
      – Posterior

   ii.  Position 'y' on the ultrasound display is toward which part of the patient?

      – Left
      – Right
      – Anterior
      – Posterior

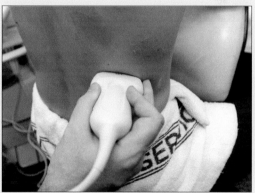

b

CHAPTER 3

## ANSWERS

 **1.** b, d

In image 'a', the operator is having to cross arms to scan and control the machine. In image 'c', the machine and patient are too far apart and the operator is having to bend over.

 **2.** b, c

In image 'a', the thumb and index finger are too far from the probe face to control it adequately. In image 'd', the wrist is bent and there are not enough fingers to spread probe forces.

 **3.** d

Vertical image from the left, showing kidney, spleen, and diaphragm.

b: axial/transverse image from the right, showing liver and kidney.
c: vertical image from the right, showing liver and kidney (note R annotation on image, and mirror image artefact).
e: Vertical image from the left, but image reversed screen left to right (patient inferior to superior), opposite to conventional orientation.

 **4a.**   i. Posterior
          ii. Superior

**4b.**   i. Posterior
          ii. Left

# Image Interpretation: Normal Ultrasound of the Chest

Claire L. Tobin

## INTRODUCTION

In healthy individuals, visualization of the lung parenchyma is not possible because the large difference in acoustic impedance (sound-conducting properties) between the chest wall and the air within the lung results in near total reflection of the ultrasound waves. Several other important structures can, however, be visualized in the normal subject when performing thoracic ultrasound.

Ultrasound images are displayed on a gray scale, and the reflected wave amplitude determines echogenicity. The strongest echo appears white (hyperechoic), while the image is black when no sound wave is reflected from the organ (anechoic). The diaphragm, pleura, and pericardium cause hyperechoic reflections on normal chest ultrasound.

Artifacts are misrepresentation of echoes in relation to the actual structures. Examples are reverberation, comet-tail, and mirror artifacts, which may be seen commonly in normal chest ultrasound (see Chapter 2). In many instances they are useful and their correct interpretation is vital for successful clinical application of pleural ultrasound.

Scanning of the lung and pleural space should be performed during quiet respiration to allow assessment of normal lung movement. In the normal upright adult patient, the lower limit of the thorax is identified ultrasonographically by locating the hemidiaphragm and liver on the right (Figure 4.1), and the hemidiaphragm and spleen on the left. During expiration the lower limit of the lungs is two costal spaces above the line of pleural reflection. The visceral and parietal pleura reach the 6th and 8th ribs, respectively, at the mid-clavicular line, the 8th and 10th ribs in the mid-axillary line, and the 10th and 12th ribs posteriorly.

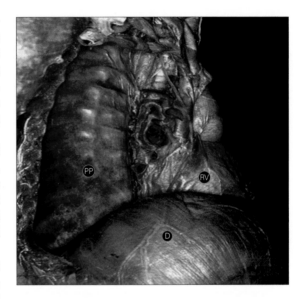

**Figure 4.1** Anatomical demonstration of the right hemithorax. Posterior chest wall dissection with intact parietal pleura (PP) and arching right hemidiaphragm (D). RV = right ventricle. (Courtesy of Dr. Helen Ward. Image provided with permission by Anatomedia, http://www.anatomedia.com)

4

# THE DIAPHRAGM AND UPPER ABDOMINAL ORGANS

Identifying the hemidiaphragm is a crucial first step in pleural ultrasound to ensure correct anatomical localization and orientation. It is best seen through the lower intercostal spaces or via the liver or spleen. Without pleural effusion the hemidiaphragm can only be partially visualized. When pleural fluid is present, it acts as an acoustic window to allow visualization of the entire course of the hemidiaphragm. The normal hemidiaphragm comprises five layers, and in thin patients with pleural effusions it is often possible to visualize all five layers.

The normal hemidiaphragm is seen as a smooth curvilinear echogenic line that is 1–2 mm thick, where the liver and spleen are seen below the hemidiaphragm on the right and left sides, respectively (Figures 4.2 and 4.3). Note should be made that the spleen often does

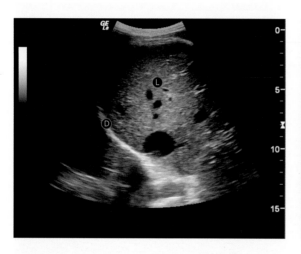

**Figure 4.2** Ultrasound appearance of liver (L) and right hemidiaphragm (D). The latter is seen as a hyperechoic curvilinear line.

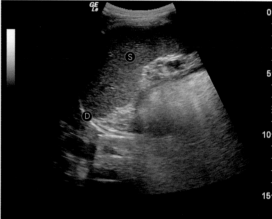

**Figure 4.3** Spleen (S) and hyperechoic left hemidiaphragm (D).

**Figure 4.4** Spleen seen inferior to lung (note movement with respiration). If the diaphragm is not visualized confidently, this may be misinterpreted as pleural fluid. 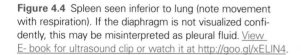 View E- book for ultrasound clip or watch it at http://goo.gl/xELlN4.

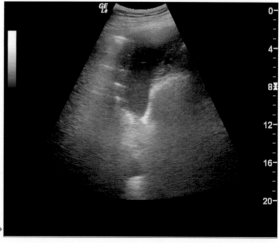

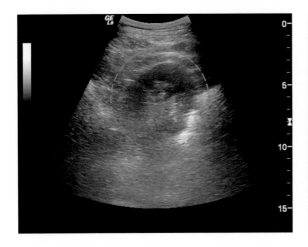

**Figure 4.5** Visualisation of right kidney (circled).

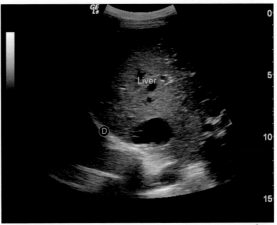

**Figure 4.6** Right hemidiaphragm movement during respiration. The diaphragm (D) contracts downward toward the liver during inspiration. View E-book for ultrasound clip or watch it at http://goo.gl/W4zqPd.

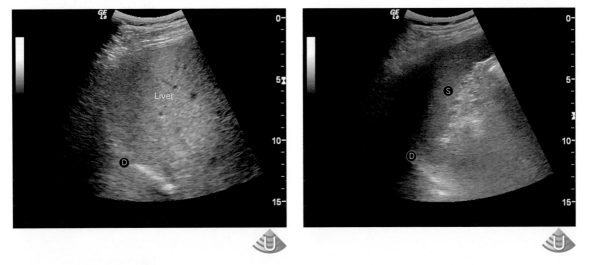

**Figures 4.7 and 4.8** Right and left hemidiaphragm (D) movement in same individual, displacing the liver (L) and spleen (S) downward during inspiration. Note the asymmetry in the diaphragm excursion between the right and left sides in this patient without pathology. View E-book for ultrasound clips or watch them at http://goo.gl/MI6Ziv and http://goo.gl/r04LHu.

not appear as dense as liver on ultrasound, which may result in it being wrongly interpreted as a fluid collection by the novice scanner (Figure 4.4—clip). For this reason, locating the diaphragm with certainty at every scan is critical. The kidney is usually visualized as an isoechoic bean-shaped structure inferior to the liver and spleen (Figure 4.5).

The normal hemidiaphragm contracts downward into the abdominal space during inspiration, usually by 5–7 cm (Figure 4.6—clip). There is wide variability in the normal movement of the diaphragm during respiration, and there is usually asymmetry in the movement of the two leaves in normal individuals[1] (Figures 4.7 and 4.8—clips).

## THE PLEURA

As the normal pleura is only 0.2–0.4 mm thick,[2] the pleural membranes are seen as a single highly echogenic horizontal line below the chest wall when using the low-frequency probe (Figure 4.9). With a high-resolution probe the parietal and visceral pleura may be seen as two distinct echogenic lines (Figure 4.10). The visceral pleura in humans is usually thicker than the parietal pleura.[3] The depth at which the pleural line is visualized will vary, depending on the thickness of the patient's chest wall, and is easily identified in relation to the adjacent rib. Beyond the pleura–lung interface, the air-filled lung does not allow further visualization of normal lung parenchyma. Hence, the ultrasound "image" of aerated lung is caused by dirty shadowing from artifact.

The respiratory movement of the lung relative to the chest wall (i.e., sliding of the visceral pleura with respiration) is seen with both probes and is called the "lung sliding" sign (Figures 4.11 and 4.12—clips). Loss of this normal sliding sign is a good indicator of underlying pleural pathology (see Chapter 7). Lung sliding is also absent in patients who have been successfully pleurodesed, at the apices in patients with severe emphysema, adjacent to large bullae, and in ventilated patients when ventilation is suspended. Scanning in M (motion) mode can be used to confirm movement at the pleural layer, with the "seashore" sign confirming the presence of lung sliding (Figure 4.13).

The pleural line may move in synchrony with cardiac pulsation. This is termed lung pulse. The movement is caused by the force of cardiac pulsation being transmitted across the lung to the visceral pleura and indicates the pleural surfaces are opposed at the site of transducer application (Figure 4.14—clip). Lung pulse is difficult to see in normally ventilated lung due to masking from lung sliding, but is easily visualized in nonventilated lung (e.g., complete atelectasis or during breath holding in normal individuals). It is more prominent in the left hemithorax.[4]

The large change in acoustic impedance at the pleura–lung interface often results in horizontal hyperechoic artifacts that are seen as a series of echogenic parallel lines equidistant from one another below the pleural line. These are termed reverberation artifacts (or A lines) (Figure 4.15) and arise when the ultrasound rebounds several times before returning to the transducer (see Chapter 2). A lines diminish in intensity with increasing distance from the pleura. Reverberation artifact may also be caused by rebounding of the ultrasound between the layers of fascia within the chest wall (Figure 4.16).

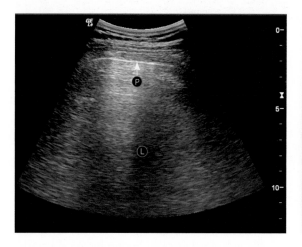

**Figure 4.9** Hyperechoic pleural line (P) and underlying normal aerated lung (L) on low-frequency probe view.

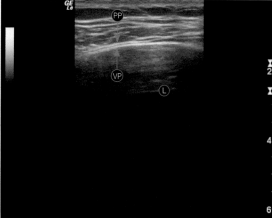

**Figure 4.10** Visceral pleura (VP) and parietal pleura (PP) seen separately with high-frequency probe. Underlying aerated lung (L).

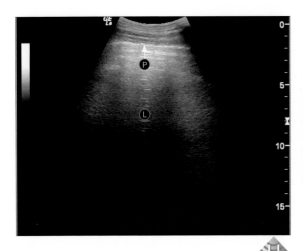

**Figure 4.11** The sliding sign: the pleura (P) is seen to slide backward and forward during normal respiration. L = underlying aerated lung. View E-book for ultrasound clip or watch it at http://goo.gl/NtWlwO.

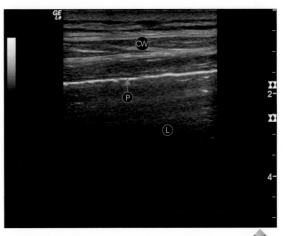

**Figure 4.12** Sliding sign visualized using high-frequency probe. P = pleura, CW = chest wall, L = underlying aerated lung. View E-book for ultrasound clip or watch it at http://goo.gl/y0HWjN.

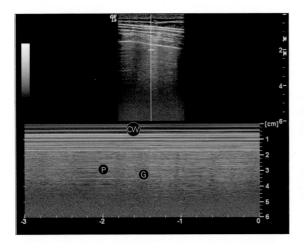

**Figure 4.13** Seashore sign in M mode, confirming lung sliding. The pleural line (P) separates two distinct patterns: the horizontal stripes of the motionless chest wall (CW) and the granular pattern (G) below this due to motion at the pleural line.

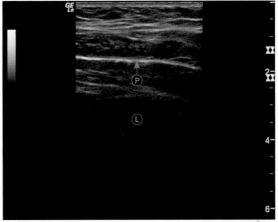

**Figure 4.14** Lung pulse sign. Pleura (P) moving in unison with cardiac pulsation due to transmission across lung (L). Confirms apposition of pleural layers at probe site. View E-book for ultrasound clip or watch it at http://goo.gl/f8iqBf.

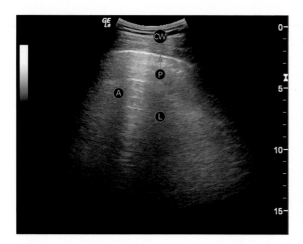

**Figure 4.15** Reverberation artifact from the pleural line (P) causing the appearance of multiple, equidistant hyperechoic lines known as A lines (A). CW = chest wall, L = aerated lung.

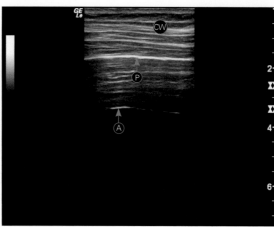

**Figure 4.16** Reverberation artifact can also be caused by the fascia planes within the chest wall (CW), producing multiple linear artifacts below the pleura (P). Note the A-line artifact from the pleura itself.

## CHEST WALL AND RIBS

The chest wall is comprised of subcutaneous tissue, muscle, and ribs. A series of echogenic layers of muscle and fascia planes are seen during surveillance of a normal chest wall (Figure 4.17).

When holding the probe against the chest wall in the horizontal/longitudinal plane (i.e., perpendicular to the ribs), the ribs will appear as curvilinear structures with posterior acoustic shadowing (Figures 4.18 and 4.19). This is caused by reflection rather than transmission of the ultrasound waves. In addition to bone, other structures that normally cause shadowing are those with calcium deposition (see Chapter 2).

When the probe is aligned directly over a rib, the anterior cortex is seen as a continuous echogenic line (Figure 4.20) that does not slide with respiration. This must not be confused with the pleural line. A break in the continuity of this line is seen in a fractured rib, and has been reported to be a very sensitive method of detecting rib fractures. It may be used to look for unsuspected rib fractures in patients with chest wall point tenderness (see Chapter 6).

The intercostal artery runs underneath the rib in the subcostal groove. However, in the first few centimeters lateral to the spine the artery is often exposed within the intercostal space (Figure 4.21). Variability of its vertical position increases with age and more cephalic rib spaces.[5] Color flow Doppler can be used to help localize intercostal vessels (Figure 4.22—clip) but needs to be used cautiously, as it produces artifact with respiratory movement, and experience is needed to interpret it. Identification of costal vessels is also dependent on other scanning parameters, such as flow velocity. It cannot be used reliably to exclude vasculature when performing an invasive procedure (Figure 4.23).

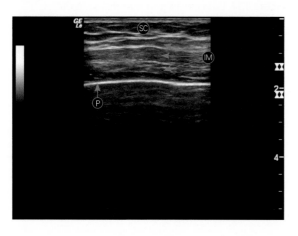

**Figure 4.17** High-frequency view of chest wall, comprised of subcutaneous tissue (SC) and underlying intercostal muscle (IM). P = pleura.

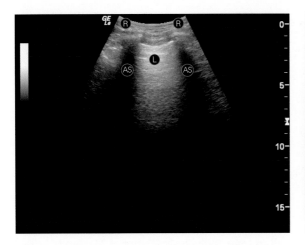

**Figure 4.18** View of the chest wall using low-frequency probe orientated in the vertical/longitudinal plane. Ribs (R) cause posterior acoustic shadowing (AS). Normal aerated lung (L).

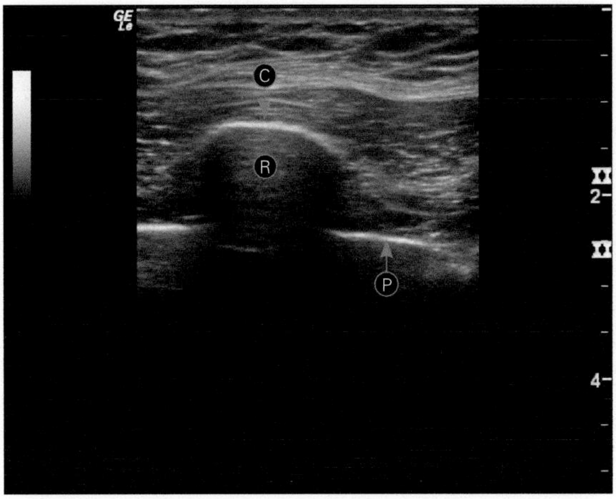

**Figure 4.19** High-frequency view of the chest wall in longitudinal plane. Rib (R) with curvilinear cortex (C) and underlying hyperechoic pleura (P).

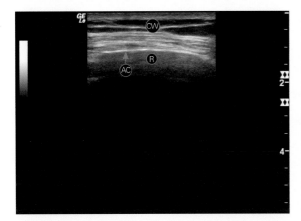

**Figure 4.20** High-frequency probe positioned directly over (and in line with) a rib (R). The anterior cortex (AC) is seen as a hyperechoic line. CW = chest wall.

**Figure 4.21** CT demonstrating the exposed nature and tortuosity of the intercostal arteries (IC) posteriorly.

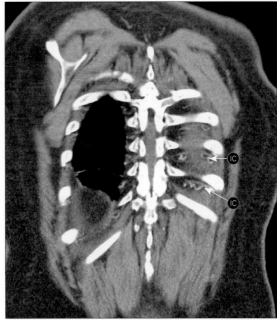

CHAPTER 4

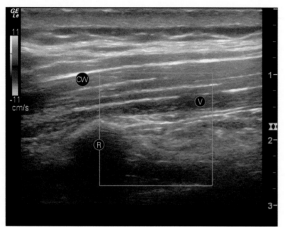

Figure 4.22 Use of color Doppler to identify intercostal vessels. Doppler should be used with caution, as identification of vasculature depends on examiner expertise and certain scan parameters. V = vessel, R = rib, CW = chest wall. View E-book for ultrasound clip or watch it at http://goo.gl/1x321t.

## HEART/MEDIASTINUM

Pleural ultrasound is not used for focused examination of the heart or mediastinal structures. However, note that the location of the left ventricle is important prior to performing an invasive procedure in the left hemithorax, as it can sit surprisingly close to the chest wall in some individuals (Figures 4.24a and b—clip). The presence of an echo-free space in this situation (from blood within the heart) must not be confused with pleural effusion.

On occasion it may also be possible to pick up pericardial pathology such as a pericardial effusion, prompting the need for echocardiogram. The mediastinal pleura cannot be visualized in the normal condition because of the interposition of aerated lung, unless using a parasternal approach.

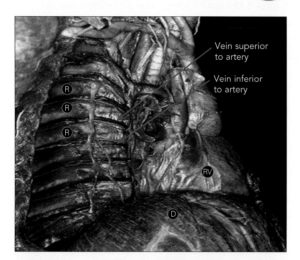

Vein superior to artery

Vein inferior to artery

Figure 4.23 Posterior chest wall dissection illustrating variability in anatomy of intercostal vessels. RV = right ventricle; D = diaphragm; R = rib. (Courtesy of Dr. Helen Ward. Image provided with permission by Anatomedia, http://www.anatomedia.com.)

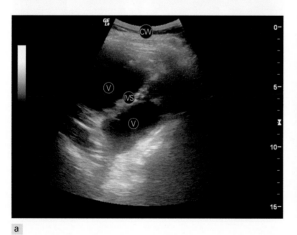

a

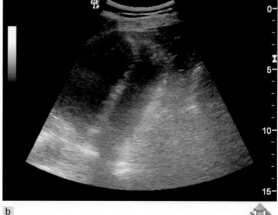

b

Figure 4.24 (a) Heart seen abutting the chest wall (CW) in a patient with dilated cardiomyopathy. Note the anechoic blood within the ventricles (V). IVS = interventricular septum. (b) Contracting heart abutting the left lateral chest wall in a patient with cardiomyopathy. View E-book for ultrasound clip or watch it at http://goo.gl/lsXGGI.

## COMMON ARTIFACTS AND SIGNS SEEN IN THE NORMAL LUNG

In addition to the reverberation artifact (or A lines) discussed above, a comet-tail artifact can also be seen in normal individuals. Comet tails are vertically oriented artifacts that originate at the pleura–lung interface. They result as a consequence of reverberation from the fluid-rich subpleural interlobular septae, which are surrounded by air. Short comet tails are seen commonly in normal lung (Figures 4.25 and 4.26—clip), and

importantly, in the presence of pneumothorax, comet-tail artifacts disappear[6] (see Chapter 7). B lines are a type of comet-tail artifact that are long, well-defined, hyperechoic lines that fan out to the edge of the screen, erase A lines, and move with respiration (Figures 4.27a and b—clip). Visualization of B lines in a healthy adult is usually confined to the last intercostal space above the diaphragm[1] and may also be seen if scanning over the area of an interlobar fissure. Certain diseases causing thickening of the interlobular septa (e.g., interstitial edema, lymphangitis, interstitial lung disease) increase

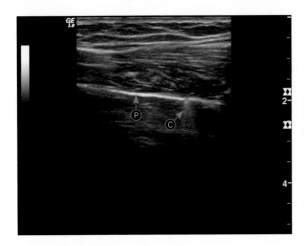

**Figure 4.25** Short comet-tail artifact (C) arising at pleura (P) –lung interface and fanning outward.

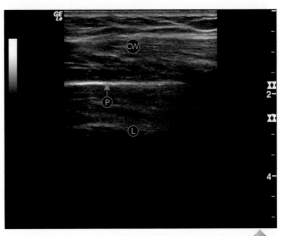

**Figure 4.26** Sliding sign with the appearance of comet tails during respiration. CW = chest wall, P = pleura, L = aerated lung. View E book for ultrasound clip or watch it at http://goo.gl/Sx9CzT.

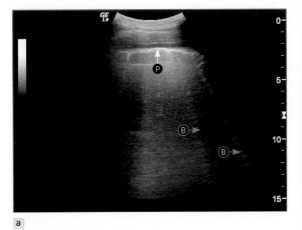

a

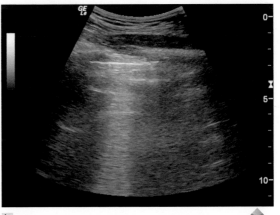

b

**Figure 4.27** (a) Echogenic B lines (B) arising at pleura (P) –lung interface and fanning outward to the edge of the screen. (b) Echogenic B lines, seen moving with respiration and fanning outward to the edge of the screen. View E-book for ultrasound clip or watch it at http://goo.gl/RpLRno.

CHAPTER 4

the number of B lines seen (often termed "lung rockets" when multiple), and the presence of ≥3 artifacts <7 mm apart is generally felt to be a realistic watershed between normal and pathological.[7]

The mirror-image artifact also needs to be recognized and understood. As the diaphragm is a strong reflector, it can cause an artifact whereby a structure (usually the liver or spleen) is seen on both sides of the diaphragm, one being a mirror image. The second (false) image is caused by reflection off the diaphragm;

the ultrasound waves take longer to travel along this path, so the probe sees the false image as being deeper, beyond the hemidiaphragm (Figure 4.28).

The "curtain" sign describes the obscuring of underlying structures by air-containing tissue. In normal subjects, the curtain sign is seen in the costophrenic angle where the upper abdominal organs are temporarily obscured during inspiration as the normal air-filled lung moves downward in front of the probe (Figures 4.29 and 4.30—clips).

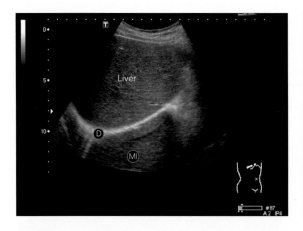

**Figure 4.28** Liver seen on both sides of the hemi-diaphragm due to mirror-image artifact. The mirror or false image (MI) is seen beyond the diaphragm due to increased transmission time of the reflected ultrasound waves off the diaphragm (D).

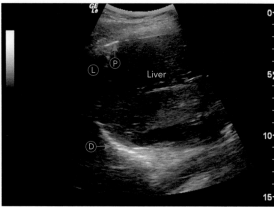

**Figure 4.29** Ultrasound clip demonstrating the curtain sign in the right hemithorax. Downward movement of aerated lung (L) causes obscuration of underlying organs during respiration. D = diaphragm, P = pleura. View E-book for ultrasound clip or watch it at http://goo.gl/zzm1sr.

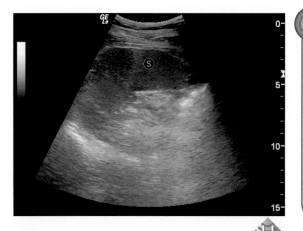

**Figure 4.30** Curtain sign in left hemithorax with intermittent obscuration of the spleen (S) by air-filled lung during respiration. View E-book for ultrasound clip or watch it at http://goo.gl/npOAMH.

## TIPS FOR CLINICAL PRACTICE

- Identify anatomic boundaries—diaphragm, chest wall, ribs, pleura, and lung.
- Identify other structures—liver, spleen, kidney, heart.
- Recognize characteristic dynamic changes—sliding sign, diaphragmatic motion, curtain sign, and lung pulse.
- Recognize and understand common normal artifacts—reverberation, mirror image, and comet tails.

# REFERENCES

1. Koh D, Burke S, Davis N, et al. Transthoracic US of the chest: clinical uses and applications. *Radiographics* 2002; 22(1):e1.

2. Vollmer I, Gayette A. Chest ultrasonography. *Arch Bronconeumol* 2010; 46(1):27–34.

3. Meuwley J, Gudinchet F. Sonography of the thoracic and abdominal walls. *J Clin Ultrasound* 2004; 32:500–10.

4. Lichtenstein DA, et al. The "lung pulse": an early ultrasound sign of complete atelectasis. *Intensive Care Med* 2003; 29(12):2187–92.

5. Helm E, Rahman N, Talakoub O, et al. Course and variation of the intercostal artery by computed tomography. *Chest* 2012; doi: 10.1378/chest.12-1285.

6. Lichtenstein D, Meziere G, Biderman P, et al. The comet tail artifact: an ultrasound sign ruling out pneumothorax. *Intensive Care Med* 1999; 25:383–88.

7. Lichtenstein D, Meziere G, Lascols N, et al. The comet-tail artefact. An ultrasound sign of alveolar-interstitial syndrome. *Am J Respir Crit Care Med* 1997; 156:1640–46.

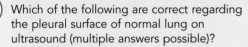

## MCQ 1

**Q** Which of the following are correct regarding the pleural surface of normal lung on ultrasound (multiple answers possible)?

a. The parietal and visceral pleura are seen as two distinct layers on low-frequency ultrasound.

b. The pleural surface may be seen to move with the heartbeat near the mediastinum.

c. The pleural surface may demonstrate B line artifacts in dependent areas.

d. The pleural surface may demonstrate B line artifacts at the interlobar fissure.

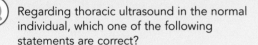

## MCQ 2

**Q** Regarding thoracic ultrasound in the normal individual, which one of the following statements are correct?

a. Ultrasound is of no clinical use in patients without pleural pathology.

b. Ultrasound can be used to reliably identify the intercostal vessels.

c. The curtain sign refers to lung sliding.

d. None of the above.

## MCQ 3

**Q** Which one of the following statements regarding comet-tail artifacts is incorrect?

a. Comet tails are a form of reverberation artifact.

b. Comet tails suggest the presence of pneumothorax at the probe site.

c. Comet tails are seen when scanning normal lung.

d. Comet tails arise from the pleural surface.

CHAPTER 4

CHAPTER 4

### MCQ 4

 **Q** Which one of the following statements regarding this image is correct?

a. The machine is scanning in B mode.

b. The presence of lung sliding is confirmed.

c. The patient has a pleural effusion.

d. The patient has a pneumothorax.

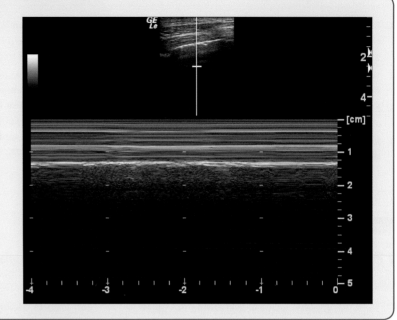

### ANSWERS

 **A** **1.** b, c, d

The visceral and parietal pleura may sometimes be seen as two separate hyperechoic lines using the high-frequency probe, not low frequency. All other statements are correct (see Chapter 4).

 **A** **2.** d

Many structures can still be identified and assessed using ultrasound in a patient without pleural pathology, including the lung, diaphragm, and chest wall. Intercostal vessels can be identified using Doppler ultrasound, but scanning parameters, operator experience and variable vessel location make it an unreliable tool to depend on. The "curtain" sign refers to the dynamic sign of upper abdominal organs becoming obscured during inspiration, as air-filled lung moves downwards in front of the probe.

 **A** **3.** b
Comet tails arise from the visceral pleural surface and therefore indicate that the two pleural layers are opposed at that site (hence no pneumothorax at the probe site). See Chapter 4 for further explanation.

 **A** **4.** b

The machine is scanning in M (motion) mode, not B mode. The different appearance above and below the bright pleural line indicates normal movement at the pleural surface (lung sliding). The stationary chest wall produces static white lines, but movement below the pleura gives a granular appearance to the image. See Chapters 4 and 7.

# Image Interpretation: Pleural Effusions

Rob Hallifax and Najib M. Rahman

## PLEURAL EFFUSION — BASIC APPEARANCE

Pleural effusion is detected at sonography as an echo-free (black) area through which deeper structures can be visualized (Figure 5.1). This is the case for so-called simple pleural effusions, meaning those that are free flowing and nonseptated. As such fluid collections normally accumulate in a gravitational distribution, small free-flowing effusions (Figure 5.2) are most readily visualized when scanning the patient in the upright position and in the most dependent part of the hemithorax, adjacent to the diaphragm and related structures. Larger effusions are usually associated with

passive collapse or atelectasis of the underlying lung (Figure 5.3a), and movement of these structures with the cardiac pulsation moving pleural fluid is typical (Figure 5.3b—clip).

The normal, aerated lung is not penetrated by ultrasound waves, and therefore the majority of the hemidiaphragm and all mediastinal structures can be difficult to visualize without the acoustic window afforded when pleural fluid is present (see Chapter 4). Pleural effusion is first recognized as an echo-free space that permits visualization of underlying structures such as

5

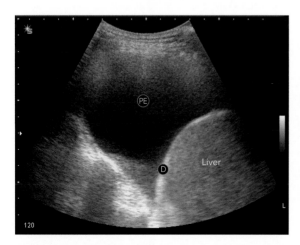

**Figure 5.1** Large pleural effusion (PE) shown by the black echo-free area. This provides an acoustic window through which the liver and entire hemidiaphragm (D) can be visualized.

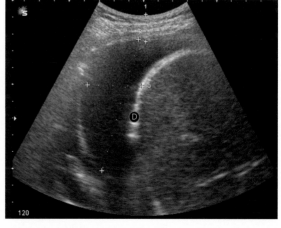

**Figure 5.2** Small basal pleural effusion. D = hemidiaphragm.

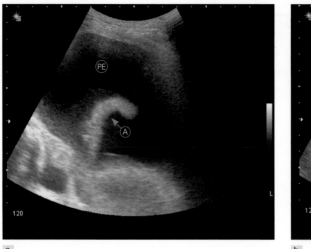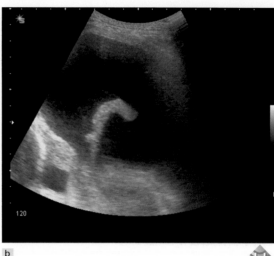

**Figure 5.3** (a) Large effusion (PE) with collapsed/atelectatic underlying lung (A). (b) The atelectatic lung can be seen moving with the transmitted cardiac pulsation. View E-book for ultrasound clip or watch it at http://goo.gl/VE9CQ8.

the diaphragm, heart, and mediastinal structures. Some caution must be applied to the scanning technique, as it is possible to achieve an entirely echo-free ultrasound field by scanning directly over a rib (Figures 5.4–5.6 —clip). The visualization of distal structures ensures that the sonographic appearance can be attributed to pleural effusion rather than poor scanning technique, and use of the depth setting on the ultrasound machine (scanning to a depth of at least 10 cm) will ensure that a mistake in identifying underlying structures is not made.

The described appearance of pleural fluid at sonography is such because fluid easily transmits ultrasound. Important differential diagnoses to bear in mind when an echo-free area is detected on thoracic ultrasound include large liver and renal cysts, ascites, stomach distended with fluid, and a dilated and poorly contracting left ventricular cavity (Figure 5.7—clip). The key to differentiating pleural fluid from these structures is identification of anatomical landmarks to ensure the fluid observed is truly in the pleural space. The most important of these structures to identify is the hemidiaphragm (see Chapters 4 and 6), which is normally a convex and moving structure located at the base of the hemithorax. However, it should be noted that the majority of patients undergoing thoracic ultrasound will be referred due to basal shadowing on a chest radiograph, for which only one diagnosis on the differential is pleural fluid. The hemidiaphragm may be paralyzed, significantly raised, or both, and hence being able to identify the hemidiaphragm in the absence of its correct position and normal movement is paramount.

## EVIDENCE FOR THORACIC ULTRASOUND IN PLEURAL FLUID DETECTION

Several studies have established thoracic ultrasound as a far more sensitive technique in pleural fluid detection than a chest radiograph.[1] Around 200 ml of pleural fluid is required before blunting of the costophrenic angle is seen on an erect chest radiograph, and pleural fluid detection using chest radiograph when the patient is supine (e.g., ventilated patients, post-trauma patients) is even more challenging.[1] While around 50 ml of pleural fluid can probably be detected on lateral decubitus chest radiograph, ultrasound has essentially replaced this radiographic modality for detection of small amounts of pleural fluid. There is, in addition, now convincing evidence that the use of thoracic ultrasound prevents inaccurate pleural puncture sites (see Chapter 1) and is likely to be the safest guide for all forms of pleural fluid intervention.

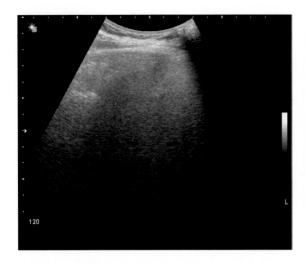

**Figure 5.4** An ultrasound image taken directly over the rib demonstrating an echo-free field with no underlying structures visible, scanning to 12 cm depth.

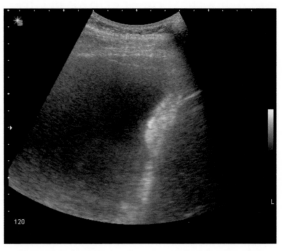

**Figure 5.5** The same patient and scan position as in Figure 5.4, but with the probe angled between, rather than over the ribs. This now demonstrates the presence of a large effusion, with the underlying structures clearly seen.

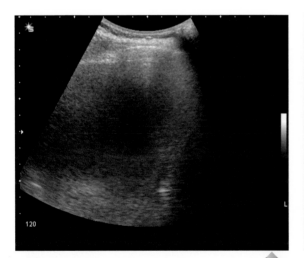

**Figure 5.6** Ultrasound clip of Figures 5.4 and 5.5 illustrating how small adjustments in probe position dramatically alter the image obtained. View E-book for ultrasound clip or watch it at http://goo.gl/iVITBK.

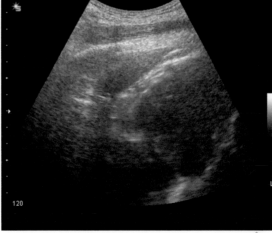

**Figure 5.7** Poorly contracting left ventricular cavity adjacent to the chest wall. The echo-free space (here due to blood within the heart) must not be confused with a pleural effusion. Note the surrounding bright pericardium. View E-book for ultrasound clip or watch it at http://goo.gl/2dvm8D.

## CALCULATION OF PLEURAL FLUID VOLUME

Several studies have assessed the use of thoracic ultrasound in estimating pleural fluid volume, with varying success.[2,3] Ultrasound is not able to consistently and accurately measure pleural fluid volume (for example, after thoracentesis), presumably due to variation in patient position and the point at which fluid is measured. Traditionally, the depth of effusion is measured from parietal pleural to underlying structure (for example, visceral pleura) at the lowest point of the hemithorax, and at the deepest part of the effusion. However, this distance will vary according to the point in the respiratory cycle, the complexity of the pleural fluid collection, as well as the fact that a given intrapleural distance represents different volumes in patients of different sizes. As a rough guide, a depth of pleural fluid of greater than 2 cm has been associated with a fluid volume of around 500 ml.[2]

The practical applicability of accurate pleural fluid volume measurement by sonographic techniques is not obvious. In cases of pleural infection, fluid should be drained dependent on the pleural fluid parameters and the clinical state of the patient.[4] In cases of effusion causing symptoms (for example, malignant pleural effusion), drainage should be aimed at symptom relief rather than being guided by the amount of fluid estimated at ultrasound.[5]

A rough practical guide to the amount of fluid present can be useful for patients in follow-up. In our practice, effusions are classified as small, moderate, or large, according to the presence of pleural fluid seen at ultrasound, with the patient in the upright position scanned posteriorly. If pleural fluid is only present in the basal hemithorax spanning one rib space, this is classified as a small effusion (Figures 5.8a and b—clip), with moderate being fluid present over two to four rib spaces, and large if the effusion occupies more than half of the hemithorax (Figures 5.9a and b—clip).

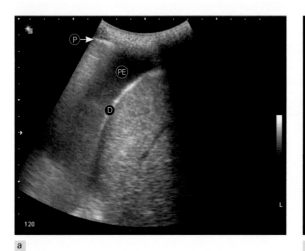
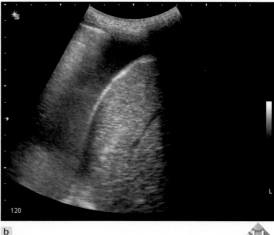

a

b

**Figure 5.8** (a) Small effusion (PE) visible above the hemidiaphragm (D). Note the echogenic pleural line (P) of normal lung above the effusion. (b) Video: normal lung movement during respiration is evident from the lung sliding sign seen above the small effusion. View E-book for ultrasound clip or watch it at http://goo.gl/R9X3u8.

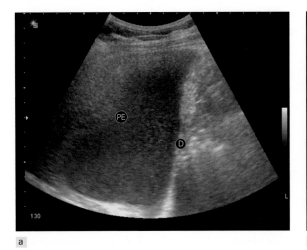
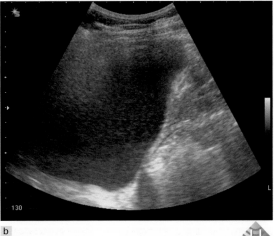

a

b

**Figure 5.9** (a) Large pleural effusion (PE) causing flattening of the hemidiaphragm (D). (b) Video: the flattened hemidiaphragm also moves poorly with respiration due to the weight of the effusion. Note: a glimpse of atelectatic lung is visible (on far left of picture) on full inspiration. View E-book for ultrasound clip or watch it at http://goo.gl/00000.

## DIFFERENTIATION OF FLUID CHARACTERISTICS

Once pleural fluid has been detected sonographically, further image interpretation and sonographic features may be used to differentiate the type, and sometimes suggest a cause, of the effusion. The amount of pleural fluid present (see above) may be estimated, but in addition, the sonographic characteristics should be interpreted.

Pleural fluid usually moves passively with cardiac pulsation and respiratory excursions (see Figure 5.3), but this effect is often difficult to visualize with 2D sonography. Color Doppler can be used to confirm the presence of pleural fluid, which moves with the cardiac pulsation (Figure 5.10—clip).[6] The color Doppler box is placed on both the effusion and the chest wall, and the color power turned up until the box is "speckling" (artifact produced by too much gain on the color Doppler). The gain is then turned down a few notches, and the movement of pleural fluid (as opposed to chest wall) assessed, which should represent cardiac pulsation. It should be noted that red and blue colors in the color Doppler scheme do not represent arterial and venous pulsation, but simply movement toward and away from the transducer.

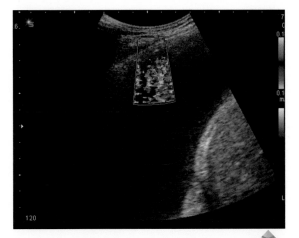

**Figure 5.10** Color Doppler can be added to 2D ultrasonography to confirm the presence of pleural fluid. The red and blue colors in the Doppler represent pleural fluid moving with the cardiac pulsation. View E-book for ultrasound clip or watch it at http://goo.gl/ugkK80.

CHAPTER 5

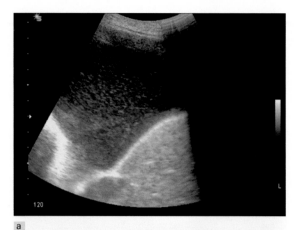

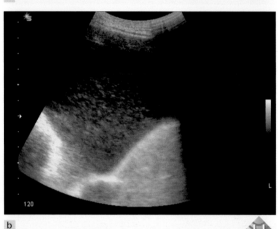

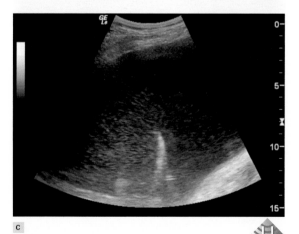

**Figure 5.11** (a) Echogenic pleural fluid. (b) Echogenic material within the effusion can be seen moving during respiration. (c) Echogenic swirling of pleural fluid. The floating and swirling echoes within the fluid are suggestive of an exudative cause of the effusion. View E-book for ultrasound clips or watch them at http://goo.gl/KNTawN and http://goo.gl/TH78CV.

This positive "fluid color" sign is diagnostic of pleural fluid moving under cardiac pulsation or respiratory movements and implies (but does not prove) the absence of significant septations preventing fluid movement.[7,8] This technique can also be used to differentiate large areas of pleural thickening (which are fluid color sign negative) from pleural fluid, and may identify consolidated lung with its characteristic vascular pattern, which on occasion may appear similar to pleural fluid in difficult to image patients (see Chapter 8).

Examination of the sonographic characteristics of detected fluid may also help in differentiating etiology. Thoracic ultrasound may differentiate "echogenic" fluid (Figure 5.11a and b—clip), where floating and swirling echoes are seen within the fluid, from "nonechogenic" fluid, whose appearance is uniform, of low attenuation throughout, and bland. Previous studies[9] suggest that the presence of echoes within the fluid is suggestive of an exudative cause of pleural effusion (where the pleura is structurally abnormal and there is usually an increased protein content of the fluid). The echoes are thought to represent collections of protein, fibrin, blood, or pus within the fluid. The identification of multiple small echoes in pleural fluid that move with cardiac and respiratory excursions is known as the "echogenic swirling" sign (Figure 5.11c—clip), and has been demonstrated to be highly sensitive for exudative causes.[10] In contrast, a nonechogenic fluid collection may be due to either transudate or exudate, and therefore this sign should be used for positive identification of exudates only where echogenic swirling is observed.

Heavily echogenic fluid, observed as increased echo signals within pleural fluid in a homogenous manner with no particular structure, has been associated with causes of effusion resulting in dense pleural fluid collections, including thick pus and hemothorax[9] (Figure 5.12a and b—clip). Empyema associated with thick pus may demonstrate multiple and brightly reflecting areas within the fluid, characteristic of air bubbles within an infected collection (Figure 5.13a and b—video). Air may also be present within an effusion in the case of bronchopleural fistula or subsequent to pleural aspiration.

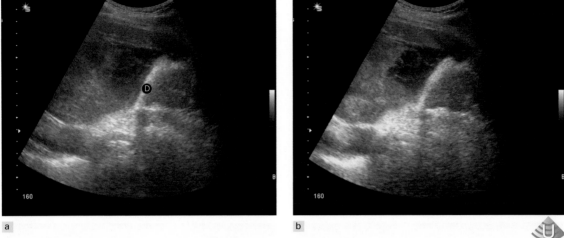

**Figure 5.12** (a) Heavily echogenic fluid with homogenously increased echo signals seen above the diaphragm (D). Causes of dense pleural fluid collections like this include thick pus and hemothorax. (b) Ultrasound clip of (a). View E-book for ultrasound clip or watch it at http://goo.gl/CGGpi7.

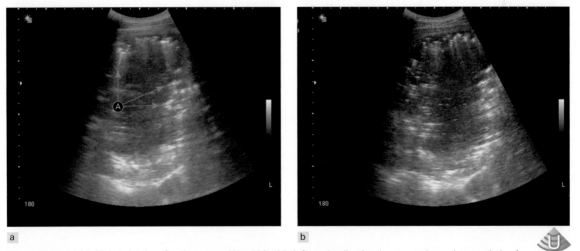

**Figure 5.13** (a) Multiple brightly reflecting areas (A) within this infected collection (empyema) are characteristic of air bubbles. (b) Ultrasound clip of (a). View E-book for ultrasound clip or watch it at http://goo.gl/ommGF3.

## SEPTATIONS

Septations are areas of fibrin within a single pleural fluid collection that partially and completely divide a single collection into many different "pockets" of fluid. This is not the same as loculation, in which there are multiple separate collections of fluid in different geographical areas of the pleural space (for example, entirely separate collections within the apical and inferior parts of the hemithorax). Whereas a 3D imaging modality (such as computed tomography (CT) or magnetic resonance imaging (MRI)) is preferred for the detection and definition of loculations, septations are exquisitely demonstrated on ultrasound and may be visible on MRI, but are in general not seen directly (only implied) on CT.

Septations are demonstrated on thoracic ultrasound as linear areas dividing pleural fluid, and may be thin and very light in echogenicity (associated with earlier, more fibrinous septations) or thicker and heavier (associated with later, more collagenous septations). The early septations (Figure 5.14a) tend to be easily deformed as a result of pleural fluid movement (Figure 5.14b—clip), whereas advanced and extensive septations (Figure 5.15a) are less so (Figure 5.15b—clip). Any effusion that is present for a prolonged period may become septated (including transudates),

but their presence is particularly associated with long-standing or previously intervened upon malignant effusions, and in infected pleural collections. There is some early evidence that the presence of sonographic septations may be associated with the need for surgical intervention during treatment for pleural infection, but these findings have not as yet been confirmed in a prospective study.[11–14]

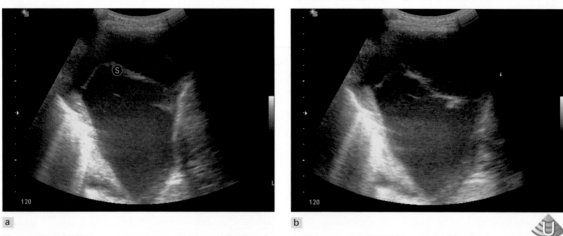

**Figure 5.14** (a) Early septations seen as thin and lightly echogenic linear strands (S) dividing pleural fluid. (b) Early septations move readily due to cardiac and respiration motion. View E-book for ultrasound clip or watch it at http://goo.gl/FUu8bB.

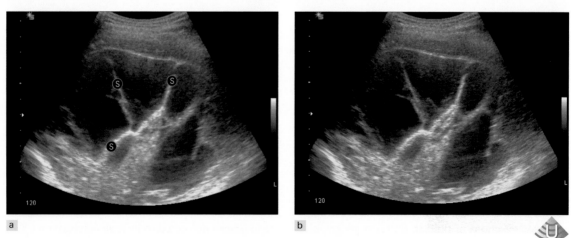

**Figure 5.15** (a) Advanced septations (S) are more collagenous, echogenic, and thicker. (b) Advanced/developed septations are less likely to move freely with cardiac and respiratory motion. View E-book for ultrasound clip or watch it at http://goo.gl/1uHBdx.

## FURTHER DIAGNOSTICS

There is now emerging data that thoracic ultrasound can be used to guide diagnosis further than the simple differentiation of transudates and exudates. The identification at thoracic ultrasound of features similar to those seen on thoracic CT[15] in malignant pleural effusion (parietal pleural thickening greater than 1 cm, nodular pleural thickening) and other features not as easily identified by CT (visceral pleural nodules (Figures 5.16a and b—clip) and diaphragmatic nodules (Figures 5.17a and b—clip) has been shown in a prospective study to diagnose malignant pleural effusion with good sensitivity and specificity.[16] Identification of parietal pleural thickening/abnormality (Figures 5.18a and b—clip) may also permit targeted biopsy to aid diagnosis.[17]

The differentiation of a small pleural effusion from pleural thickening can be challenging. Pleural thickening can be anechoic or hypoechoic, and therefore the sole presence of an echo-free space between the parietal and visceral pleura does not guarantee the presence of pleural fluid. In this case, use of color Doppler may be useful, with pleural fluid displaying a

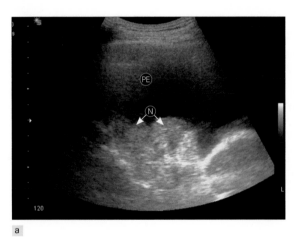
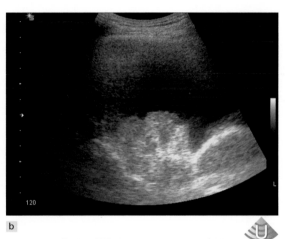

**Figure 5.16** (a) Visceral pleural nodules (N) seen easily through the pleural effusion (PE). (b) Ultrasound clip of (a). View E-book for ultrasound clip or watch it at http://goo.gl/PcR0JJ.

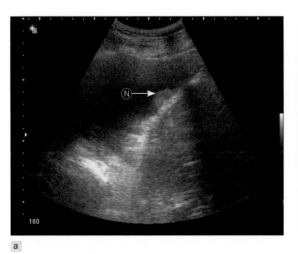
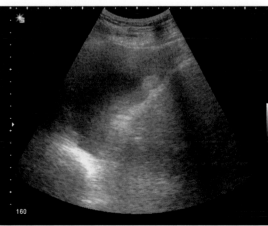

**Figure 5.17** (a) Diaphragmatic nodule (N). (b) Ultrasound clip of (a). View E-book for ultrasound clip or watch it at http://goo.gl/3WPHFE.

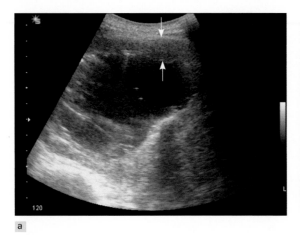
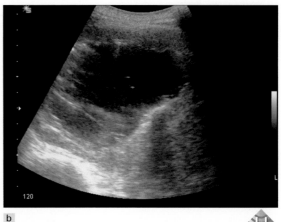

**Figure 5.18** (a) Parietal pleural thickening, seen here as smooth thickening between the arrows. (b) Ultrasound clip of (a). View E-book for ultrasound clip or watch it at http://goo.gl/QwHnJJ.

positive "color fluid" sign (see above), whereas pleural thickening will not. In addition, areas of pleural thickening may demonstrate a vascular pattern more similar to a vascularized tissue than the chaotic color sign observed with pleural fluid.

The appearance of pneumothorax at thoracic ultrasound is described in detail in Chapter 7, but the presence of both free fluid and air (hydropneumothorax) produces a particular appearance. In this case, fluid is seen (usually basally according to gravity) as

an echo-free space through which distal structures can be appreciated, as in all effusions. Adjacent to the fluid is the air that produces reflection artifact and through which distal structures cannot be appreciated. Although the appearance of the pneumothorax may be mistaken for lung, the pneumothorax lacks the normal pleural sliding sign (see Chapter 4) and, importantly, will move in a chaotic manner in line with the cardiac and respiratory excursions (Figure 5.19—clip).

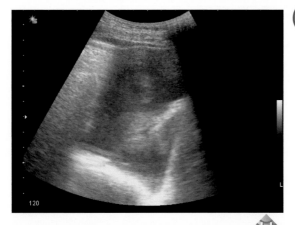

**Figure 5.19** Typical appearance of a hydro-pneumothorax. Pleural effusion is seen basally (with the intermittent appearance of lung in this case), and free air in the pleural space above the effusion is distinguished from normal lung by the absence of normal lung sliding and movement in a chaotic manner. View E-book for ultrasound clip or watch it at http://goo.gl/Y45kOR.

### TIPS FOR CLINICAL PRACTICE

- Orientate yourself by first identifying the diaphragm.
- Fluid appears black (echo-free).
- Color Doppler can help confirm the presence of pleural effusions by showing movement with cardiac pulsation.
- Identify underlying structures—heart, mediastinal structures—and look for consolidated/atelectatic lung.
- Echogenic swirling sign is highly sensitive for exudative causes of effusions.

# REFERENCES

1. Eibenberger KL, Dock WI, Ammann ME, Dorffner R, Hormann MF, Grabenwoger F. Quantification of pleural effusions: sonography versus radiography. *Radiology* 1994; 191(3):681–684.

2. Balik M, Plasil P, Waldauf P, Pazout J, Fric M, Otahal M, et al. Ultrasound estimation of volume of pleural fluid in mechanically ventilated patients. *Intensive Care Med* 2006; 32(2):318–321.

3. Roch A, Bojan M, Michelet P, Romain F, Bregeon F, Papazian L, et al. Usefulness of ultrasonography in predicting pleural effusions > 500 mL in patients receiving mechanical ventilation. *Chest* 2005; 127(1):224–232.

4. Davies HE, Davies RJ, Davies CW. Management of pleural infection in adults: British Thoracic Society Pleural Disease Guideline 2010. *Thorax* 2010; 65(Suppl 2):ii41–ii53.

5. Roberts ME, Neville E, Berrisford RG, Antunes G, Ali NJ. Management of a malignant pleural effusion: British Thoracic Society Pleural Disease Guideline 2010. *Thorax* 2010; 65(Suppl 2):ii32–ii40.

6. Wu RG, Yuan A, Liaw YS, Chang DB, Yu CJ, Wu HD, et al. Image comparison of real-time gray-scale ultrasound and color Doppler ultrasound for use in diagnosis of minimal pleural effusion. *Am J Respir Crit Care Med* 1994; 150(2):510–514.

7. Wu RG, Yang PC, Kuo SH, Luh KT. "Fluid color" sign: a useful indicator for discrimination between pleural thickening and pleural effusion. *J Ultrasound Med* 1995; 14(10):767–769.

8. Marks WM, Filly RA, Callen PW. Real-time evaluation of pleural lesions: new observations regarding the probability of obtaining free fluid. *Radiology* 1982; 142(1):163–164.

9. Yang PC, Luh KT, Chang DB, Wu HD, Yu CJ, Kuo SH. Value of sonography in determining the nature of pleural effusion: analysis of 320 cases. *AJR Am J Roentgenol* 1992; 159(1):29–33.

10. Chian CF, Su WL, Soh LH, Yan HC, Perng WC, Wu CP. Echogenic swirling pattern as a predictor of malignant pleural effusions in patients with malignancies. *Chest* 2004; 126(1):129–134.

11. Chen CH, Chen W, Chen HJ, Yu YH, Lin YC, Tu CY, et al. Transthoracic ultrasonography in predicting the outcome of small-bore catheter drainage in empyemas or complicated parapneumonic effusions. *Ultrasound Med Biol* 2009; 35(9):1468–1474.

12. Chen KY, Liaw YS, Wang HC, Luh KT, Yang PC. Sonographic septation: a useful prognostic indicator of acute thoracic empyema. *J Ultrasound Med* 2000; 19(12):837–843.

13. Ramnath RR, Heller RM, Ben-Ami T, Miller MA, Campbell P, Neblett WW III, et al. Implications of early sonographic evaluation of parapneumonic effusions in children with pneumonia. *Pediatrics* 1998; 101(1 Pt 1):68–71.

14. Shankar S, Gulati M, Kang M, Gupta S, Suri S. Image-guided percutaneous drainage of thoracic empyema: can sonography predict the outcome? *Eur Radiol* 2000; 10(3):495–499.

15. Leung AN, Muller NL, Miller RR. CT in differential diagnosis of diffuse pleural disease. *AJR Am J Roentgenol* 1990; 154(3):487–492.

16. Qureshi NR, Rahman NM, Gleeson FV. Thoracic ultrasound in the diagnosis of malignant pleural effusion. *Thorax* 2008; 64(2):139–143.

17. Diacon AH, Schuurmans MM, Theron J, Schubert PT, Wright CA, Bolliger CT. Safety and yield of ultrasound-assisted transthoracic biopsy performed by pulmonologists. *Respiration* 2004; 71(5):51–522.

## MCQ 1

**Q** What is the main feature shown in this ultrasound image?

a. Liver with cysts.

b. Normal lung.

c. Heavily septated pleural fluid.

d. Consolidated lung.

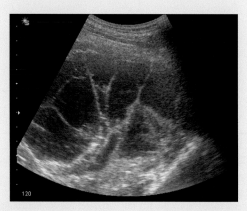

## MCQ 2

**Q** Color Doppler can be useful in confirming pleural fluid by:

a. Clarifying that no air is present in the pleural space.

b. Looking for air movement within the fluid.

c. Assessing normal diaphragmatic movement.

d. Checking for movement of the fluid in association with cardiac pulsation.

## MCQ 3

**Q** True or false? When an effusion is present you will not see the normal "lung sliding" sign.

## MCQ 4

**Q** Name the structures labeled x, y, z, and the arrow in this image.

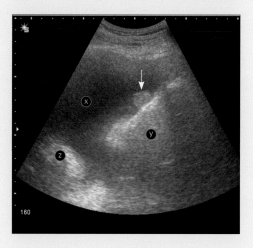

## ANSWERS

**A** 1. c

**A** 2. d  See Chapter 5.

**A** 3. False

This depends on the size of the effusion. Unless the lung is completely collapsed, you will usually see normal sliding lung above an effusion.

**A** 4. x = pleural effusion, y = liver,
z = collapsed/atelectatic lung,
arrow = diaphragmatic nodule.

# Image Interpretation: Related Thoracic Structures

John M. Wrightson and Edward T. Fysh

## INTRODUCTION

Thoracic ultrasound is an excellent imaging modality for recognizing a variety of thoracic pathologies in addition to pleural fluid. Frequently encountered abnormalities affect the lungs (atelectasis, consolidation, abscess, and tumor), heart (pericardial effusion), diaphragm (nodules, paresis/paralysis and paradoxical motion), and abdomen (ascites and hepatic metastases). Recognition of such abnormalities is essential, and may:

- Support a suspected diagnosis (e.g., malignancy when diaphragmatic nodules or likely hepatic metastases are seen).
- Suggest an alternative diagnosis (e.g., finding an unexpected pericardial effusion when imaging pleural effusions).
- Prevent injudicious pleural intervention (e.g., identify collapse/consolidation as the cause of radiographic opacity, rather than pleural effusion).

Review of any preexisting imaging, particularly cross-sectional, prior to ultrasound is essential in predicting likely findings and can aid image interpretation. This is particularly important for the trainee sonographer, who may otherwise fail to detect a lesion or misinterpret abnormalities.

## LUNG

Ultrasound is unable to image normal lung due to wave reflection at the pleural stripe caused by impedance mismatch between soft tissues and aerated lung. Lung becomes sonographically visible when pathological processes replace air within the subpleural parenchyma. Common causes of nonaerated lung include atelectasis (both passive and due to proximal obstruction), consolidation, or tumor.

### Atelectatic lung
Passive atelectasis
One of the most frequently encountered abnormalities is passive atelectasis, which frequently accompanies a moderate or large pleural effusion. This produces a characteristic "hockey stick" appearance, and improves sonographically after a therapeutic pleural aspiration.

6

Features (Figures 6.1a and b—clip, and 6.2):

- Iso/hyperechoic lung, which has significant *volume loss* and is often triangular or hockey stick-shaped and is usually surrounded by pleural fluid. (Echogenicity is conventionally defined with respect to the echogenicity of the liver.)
- Atelectatic lung has a discernable *internal structure* and *clear margins*.
- Lung movement often accompanies cardiac pulsation.

## Obstructive atelectasis

This is identified as nonaerated collapsed lung with associated minor pleural effusion. If the proximal cause is sufficiently large (pulmonary tumor—usually larger than 3 cm, or large volume lymphadenopathy), it may be seen through the atelectatic lung.

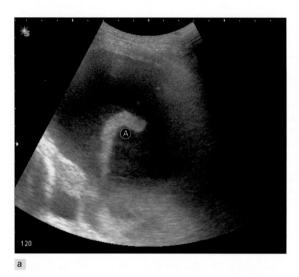
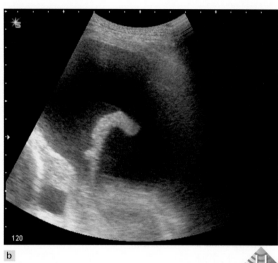

a      b

**Figure 6.1** (a) Hockey stick-shaped atelectatic lung (A) surrounded by hypoechoic pleural fluid. (b) Hockey stick-shaped atelectatic lung (demonstrating transmitted cardiac pulsation) surrounded by hypoechoic pleural fluid. View E-book for ultrasound clip or watch it at http://goo.gl/b6KLgB.

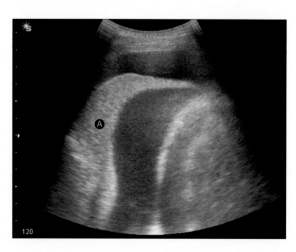

**Figure 6.2** Atelectatic lung (A) surrounded by hypoechoic pleural fluid.

## Consolidated lung

During the acute "hepatization" phase of lobar or segmental pneumonia, inflammatory cells and exudate replace air within the lung. When this consolidation abuts the pleura, it is visible at ultrasound and appearances may mimic the liver. As pneumonia resolves, the lung becomes increasingly aerated, and the consolidation becomes less distinct due to increasing air artifacts. Ultrasound often underestimates the extent of pneumonia, as it fails to detect consolidation not in continuity with the pleura. In particular, patchy multifocal consolidation is often poorly visualized.

Frequently seen features include (Figures 6.3a and b—clip, 6.4, and 6.5—clip)[1–3]:

- Hypo- or hyperechoic nonaerated lung *without volume loss*.
- Visible detail within the lung (often similar to liver) with irregular, indistinct margins.

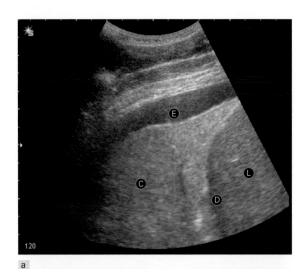

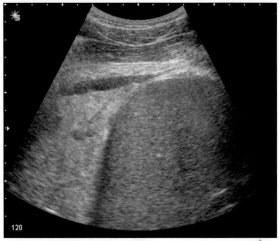

**Figure 6.3** (a) Consolidated lung (C) adjacent to hemidiaphragm (D) and liver (L). A paucity of air speckles and bronchograms raises the possibility of bronchial obstruction (by mucus or tissue). There is also a small overlying anechoic parapneumonic effusion (E). (b) Consolidated lung, with visible vasculature and a paucity of air speckles and bronchograms raising the possibility of bronchial obstruction (by mucus or tissue). Other visible features include hemidiaphragm, liver, and a small anechoic parapneumonic effusion. View E-book for ultrasound clip or watch it at http://goo.gl/QM9MfG.

CHAPTER 6

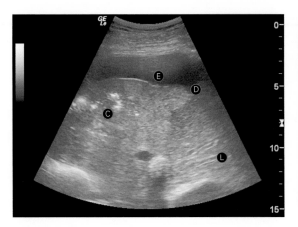

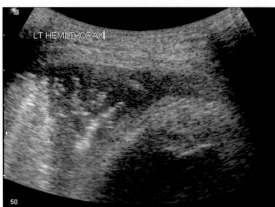

**Figure 6.4** Consolidated lung (C) with visible air speckles adjacent to hemidiaphragm (D), liver (L), and a small overlying anechoic parapneumonic effusion (E).

**Figure 6.5** Resolving pneumonia—prominent air bronchograms within a small area of consolidation. View E-book for ultrasound clip or watch it at http://goo.gl/1rOKNM.

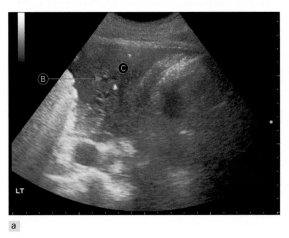

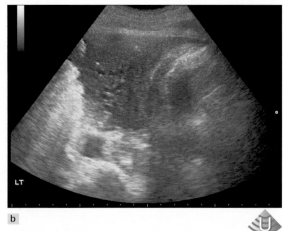

a

b

**Figure 6.6** (a) Anechoic fluid bronchograms (B) within consolidated lung (C). (b) Fluid bronchograms within consolidated lung. View E-book for ultrasound clip or watch it at http://goo.gl/NFPFO6.

- *Branching linear hypo- or anechoic structures* within consolidation representing either fluid-filled bronchi or vessels (Figure 6.6a and b—clip). Differentiation is possible with color Doppler (Figure 6.7—clip); bronchial walls also tend to be thicker with increased echogenicity.
- *Bright speckles* are caused by air, either within bronchi (appearing as branching bright linear structures—sonographic air bronchograms) or trapped within the parenchyma (appearing as small lenticular echoes).[4]
- *Abscesses* (see below).

While pneumonia is the most common cause of consolidation, other causes (e.g., pulmonary emboli, hemorrhage, vasculitis, and malignancies such as minimally invasive adenocarcinoma and invasive adenocarcinoma [previously classified as bronchoalveolar cell carcinoma] and lymphoma) may give similar appearances and should be considered in the differential diagnosis, particularly given an atypical history.

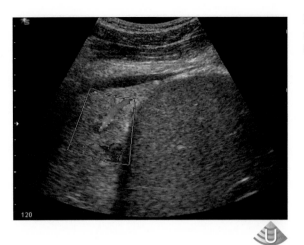

**Figure 6.7** Increased vascularity within consolidated lung, demonstrated using color Doppler. <u>View E-book for ultrasound clip or watch it at http://goo.gl/10ViJU.</u>

## Lung abscesses

These are usually seen associated with pneumonia and vary in size and number. It is not uncommon to detect small abscesses using ultrasound that would otherwise fail to be detected on chest x-ray, or suspected clinically. Ultrasound may be used to aspirate abscess pus for microbiological culture when the abscess is sonographically visible (i.e., in continuity with the pleura or surrounded by subpleural consolidation).

Pulmonary abscesses abutting the pleura may be difficult to differentiate from empyema on ultrasound, even in the context of adjacent pneumonia. If there is doubt, and differentiation is important clinically, computed tomography (CT) will help differentiate these two diagnoses.

Features[5]:

- *Rounded or oval hypo/anechoic* structures often found within consolidated lung.
- May contain *echogenic speckles* (if gas forming) and septations.
- Frequently demonstrate *posterior acoustic enhancement* (structures distal to abscess appear brighter) due to augmented ultrasound wave transmission through the abscess fluid.

## Tumors

Subpleural lung tumors may be visualized (and sampled) using ultrasound. Parietal pleural infiltration (indicating a T3 tumor) may be suggested by a loss of pleural sliding and confirmed when there is visible chest wall infiltration. Importantly, the demonstration of sliding confirms a T2 tumor, but only the demonstration of extrapleural fat or deeper invasion is definitive proof of T3 stage, as non-malignant adhesions may result in a lack of pleural sliding.

Proximal lung tumors are only visible if associated with obstructive pneumonitis or atelectasis, which allows a sonographic "window" through the lung to the tumor.[6] Due to bronchial obstruction, this consolidation is associated with a relative lack of air bronchograms or parenchymal air speckles, while having prominent fluid bronchograms.

Features of lung tumors (Figures 6.8a and b—clip):

- *Well-defined*, often *hypoechoic*, lesions frequently accompanied by *anechoic necrotic areas.*
- May have *strong peripheral vascularization*, occasionally with a tortuous "corkscrew pattern" due to neovascularization[7].
- Parietal pleural surface may be irregular, and associated with invasion of adjacent structures[8,9].
- Disruption of normal architecture of lung, particularly vessels and bronchi.

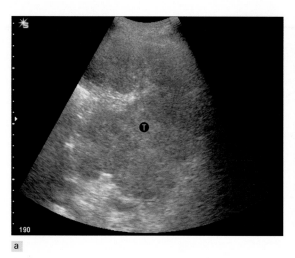 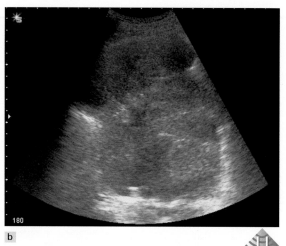

**Figure 6.8** (a) Heterogeneous hypoechoic lung tumor (T) with disruption of normal parenchymal architecture. (b) Heterogeneous hypoechoic lung tumor with disruption of normal parenchymal architecture. View E-book for ultrasound clip or watch it at http://goo.gl/x12UxW.

## Tethering

Previous or ongoing pleural insults (such as pleural infection, chemical pleurodesis, and malignancy) can cause adherence between parts of the visceral and parietal pleura, leading to a tethered lung (Figures 6.9 and 6.10—clip). It is particularly important to detect such abnormalities to avoid lung trauma during chest tube insertion or pleural fluid aspiration.

## Pulmonary emboli

Some physicians advocate the use of thoracic ultrasound in detecting pulmonary emboli,[10] but this has not gained widespread acceptance due to the high sensitivity and specificity of modern CT pulmonary angiography. Peripheral emboli often cause ultrasound-detectable parenchymal changes, but these are rather nonspecific. Large central emboli may not cause any detectable abnormalities. Differentiation between pulmonary emboli and pneumonia can be challenging, particularly as emboli start to resolve.

Features:

- *Wedge-shaped* or *rounded consolidation* caused by alveolar edema and red blood cells.
- Consolidation is initially *homogeneous* and *hypoechoic*, with relative lack of air artifacts (in contrast to pneumonia).

- Subsequently, consolidation becomes increasingly *heterogeneous* with a visible central *hyperechoic bronchus*.
- Acutely, color Doppler may demonstrate *poor blood flow*.
- Emboli are commonly accompanied by a *small pleural effusion*.
- Large/multiple emboli may cause *right ventricular strain*. Signs include a disproportionately *large right ventricle* (compared to the left), a *poorly contracting right ventricle*, and *intraventricular septal bowing* to the left. The inferior vena cava may also be enlarged, having minimal variation with respiration.

While ultrasound features may suggest pulmonary emboli, a CT pulmonary angiogram is strongly recommended to confirm ultrasound findings. Furthermore, given its frequent failure to detect central emboli, ultrasound should not be relied upon to exclude pulmonary emboli.

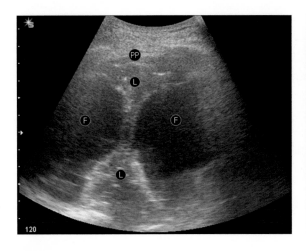

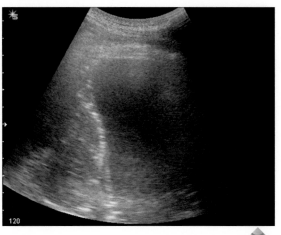

**Figure 6.9** Atelectatic lung (L) that is tethered to the parietal pleura (PP) and is surrounded by hypoechoic pleural fluid (F).

**Figure 6.10** Atelectatic lung that is tethered to the parietal pleura and is surrounded by hypo-echoic pleural fluid. View E-book for ultrasound clip or watch it at http://goo.gl/db1eiN.

## Pulmonary edema and other alveolar/interstitial changes

Normally aerated lung is associated with the following artifacts (also see Chapter 4):

- Horizontal reverberation artifacts (A lines) caused by impedance mismatch at the pleural stripe. These are seen as multiple equally spaced horizontal lines lying deep (and parallel) to the pleural stripe, which diminish in echogenicity with increasing depth.
- Occasional comet-tail artifacts (B lines) in dependent areas, caused by fluid-filled interlobular septae. On imaging, these are seen as near-vertical lines radiating out from the pleural stripe and extending to the bottom of the image.

Pathology of the alveoli and interstitium (e.g., pulmonary edema, ARDS, and interstitial lung disease) *increases the number of comet tails*, which also become visible in nondependent locations (see Chapter 10). These changes are considered significant when more than three comet tails are seen in two different ultrasound fields obtained from the same hemithorax.[11–14] While being nonspecific, increased comet tails may have clinical utility in defined situations—one study suggested that a lack of comet tails at the anterior chest can rule out cardiogenic pulmonary edema[15]; another study found that abnormal comet tails allowed differentiation between pulmonary edema and COPD exacerbation during acute respiratory failure.[16]

## DIAPHRAGM

In health, the characteristic dome-shaped diaphragm is poorly visualized due to overlying aerated lung in the costophrenic recesses, although partial views may be obtained by angling the probe upward and scanning through the liver or spleen. In the presence of pleural fluid, good views are possible and *five alternating hyper- and hypoechoic layers* may be visualized with high-frequency transducers. An artifactual "diaphragmatic gap" is occasionally seen, appearing as an apparent defect in the diaphragm. This is due to ultrasound wave refraction (causing poor return of the ultrasound beam to the transducer); repositioning the probe will confirm diaphragmatic integrity.

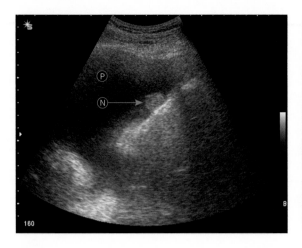

**Figure 6.11** Diaphragmatic nodularity (N) in association with a large pleural effusion (P).

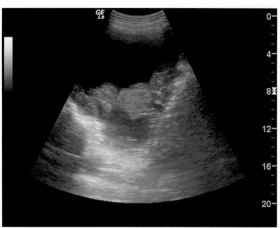

**Figure 6.12** Extensive diaphragmatic and visceral pleural nodularity consistent with malignancy (see corresponding CT—Figure 6.13). View E-book for ultrasound clip or watch it at http://goo.gl/MpTrdn.

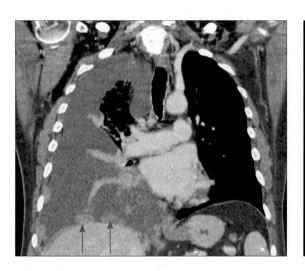

**Figure 6.13** CT corresponding to Figure 6.12 showing extensive diaphragmatic (arrows) and parietal pleural nodularity (visceral nodularity not demonstrated on this section).

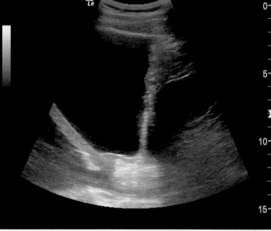

**Figure 6.14** Flattened and thickened left hemi-diaphragm associated with a large pleural effusion. View E-book for ultrasound clip or watch it at http://goo.gl/NS9ORi.

The diaphragmatic pleural surface is a common site of metastases, which appear as *nodules* or larger masses and may cause *disruption of the diaphragmatic layers* (Figures 6.11, 6.12—clip, and 6.13). Muscular diaphragmatic contraction can cause wavelike ridges in the diaphragm that may be misinterpreted as nodules, and physicians should take care not to misinterpret such findings.

Large pleural effusions may cause *flattening or inversion* of the diaphragmatic dome (Figures 6.14—clip, 6.15—clip, and 6.16a–c). Such findings are usually associated with significant dyspnea; removal of fluid sufficient to restore diaphragmatic configuration usually causes significant symptomatic benefit.

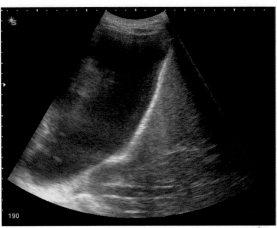

**Figure 6.15** Diaphragmatic inversion in association with a large pleural effusion, restricting diaphragmatic excursion. View E-book for ultrasound clip or watch it at http://goo.gl/44gN7n.

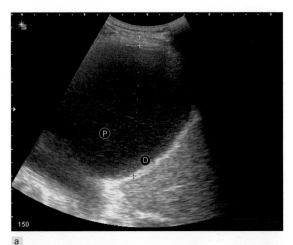

a

**Figure 6.16** (a) Inverted right hemidiaphragm (D) caused by a large echogenic pleural effusion (P). (b) Coronal CT image of grossly inverted right hemidiaphragm (D) caused by a large pleural effusion (P). (c) Post-drainage coronal CT image in same patient showing restored curvature of the right hemidiaphragm (D).

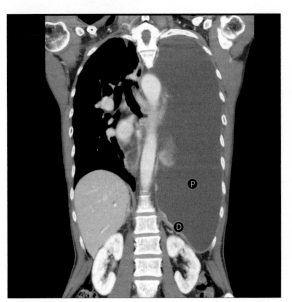

b

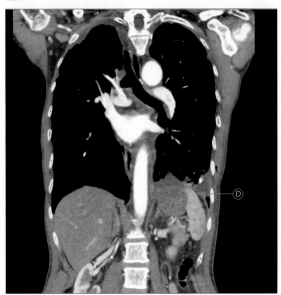

c

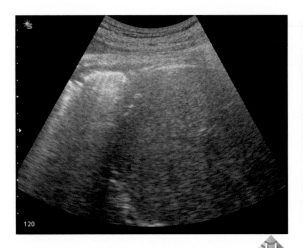

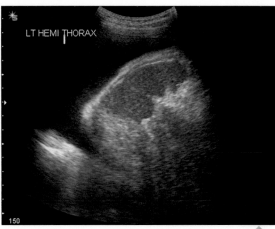

**Figure 6.17** Paralyzed right hemidiaphragm that was also noted to be markedly elevated. View E-book for ultrasound clip or watch it at http://goo.gl/25bON8.

**Figure 6.18** Poorly moving left hemidiaphragm adjacent to pleural fluid. View E-book for ultrasound clip or watch it at http://goo.gl/3D4B93.

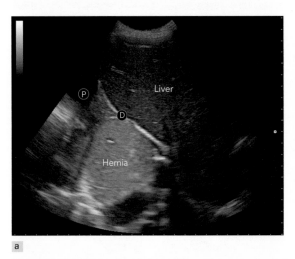

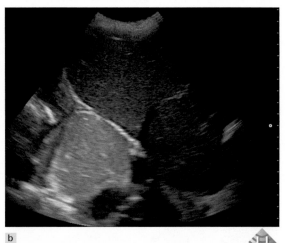

**Figure 6.19** (a) Hiatus hernia (containing echogenic stomach contents) seen adjacent to diaphragm (D) and liver in right hemithorax. Pleural fluid (P) is also visible. (b) Echogenic swirling visible within hiatus hernia, adjacent to hemidiaphragm and liver. View E-book for ultrasound clip or watch it at http://goo.gl/H3n6y7.

Ultrasound is well suited to the assessment of possible *diaphragmatic paralysis*, allowing real-time visualization of diaphragmatic motion.[17,18] It is useful in differentiating between paralysis and other causes of an apparently elevated hemidiaphragm (including hepato/splenomegaly, subpulmonary effusion, and subphrenic abscess).

Physiologically, during inspiration the peripheral muscular part of the diaphragm contracts and becomes shorter and thicker, pulling the diaphragmatic dome downward. Investigation of diaphragmatic motion may be assisted by asking the patient to sniff. Diaphragmatic paralysis is associated with a *raised hemidiaphragm*, which moves either poorly or *paradoxically* (i.e., moving upward on inspiration) (Figures 6.17—clip and 6.18—clip).

Other diaphragmatic pathology, such as herniae, may be also be encountered at ultrasound. A large hiatus hernia may mimic an echogenic pleural space, risking inappropriate chest tube insertion (Figure 6.19a and b—clip).

## HEART

Detailed echocardiography requires formal training and is beyond the scope of this book. Nevertheless, it is important for a physician to be competent in:

- Locating the heart.
- Measuring the distance between the chest wall and the pericardium.
- Making a basic assessment of significant cardiac pathology.

While the standard curvilinear ultrasound probe is not used for detailed echocardiography, it provides reasonable images of the heart, particularly in the presence of a left-sided pleural effusion that provides an "acoustic window" through which the heart may be visualized (Figures 6.20 and 6.21—clip). Where available, a phased-array echocardiography probe (which has a smaller footprint) may provide better views through narrow intercostal spaces.

The standard echocardiographic views are left and right parasternal, apical, and subxiphoid or subcostal views. However, the easiest way to visualize the heart in the setting of a pleural effusion is with the patient sat upright leaning slightly to the left, with the probe held as close to the cardiac apex as possible. A large free-flowing left pleural effusion, however, enables visualization of the heart over most of the hemithorax, enabling physicians to undertake pleural procedures without risk of causing cardiac damage.

The heart's dense hyperechoic musculature surrounding anechoic chambers undergoing rhythmic contraction is usually easily visible; however, color Doppler may provide further confirmation where pleural anatomy is very complex. A subxiphoid view, avoiding the pleural space, may be helpful in this setting and is helpful when looking for pericardial effusions and right heart pathology.

CHAPTER 6

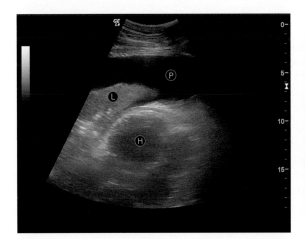

**Figure 6.20** Left pleural effusion (P) providing an acoustic window to the heart (H) and atelectatic lung (L).

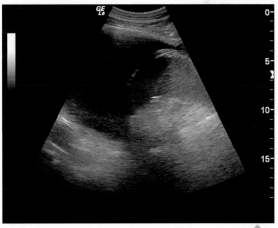

**Figure 6.21** Pleural effusion providing an acoustic window to the heart. Contracting hyper-echoic myocardium is seen surrounding hypoechoic blood. View E-book for ultrasound clip or watch it at http://goo.gl/lLqpw7.

## Pericardial effusion

This is not uncommon in association with pleural malignancy, and should always be sought in patients with pleural effusions, particularly when disproportionately dyspnoeic (Figures 6.22a and b—clip, and 6.23—clip). A large chronic pericardial effusion may be associated with remarkably few symptoms (e.g., chronic pericardial effusion in renal failure), while conversely, a relatively small acute effusion can be life threatening. Having detected a pericardial effusion, physicians are encouraged to obtain formal echocardiography and to liaise with cardiology colleagues to adequately interpret findings and ensure follow-up.

## Cardiac tamponade

Cardiac tamponade is a life-threatening emergency that can be diagnosed on ultrasound with an accuracy of 97.5% by appropriately trained non-cardiology physicians.[19] While tamponade is classically associated with the triad of low blood pressure, distended neck veins, and muffled heart sounds, some patients may present subacutely with dyspnea and pleural effusions, and have incipient tamponade detected on ultrasound.

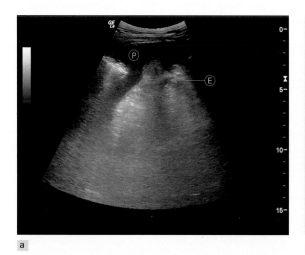

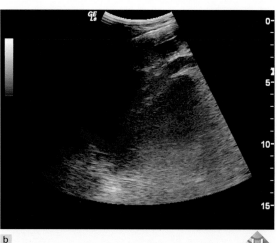

**Figure 6.22** (a) Pleural effusion (P) adjacent to a small pericardial effusion (E). (b) Left pleural effusion seen surrounding a small pericardial effusion. Apparent pericardial nodularity is seen due to fatty tissue—this is a common finding, and should be interpreted with caution. View E-book for ultrasound clip or watch it at http://goo.gl/vRcuoM.

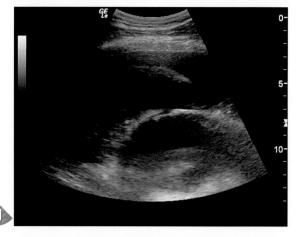

**Figure 6.23** Large pericardial effusion adjacent to pleural fluid and atelectatic lung. Such findings should prompt a formal echocardiogram and clinical assessment for possible cardiac tamponade. View E-book for ultrasound clip or watch it at http://goo.gl/ch22nY.

CHAPTER 6

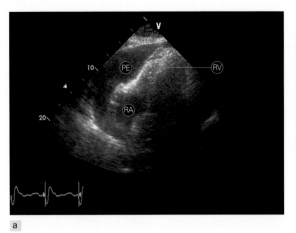
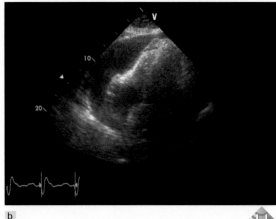

**Figure 6.24** (a) Large pericardial effusion (PE) causing compression of the right atrium (RA) and diastolic collapse of the right ventricle (RV). (b) Apical view of a rapidly contracting heart and a large pericardial effusion (PE) causing compression of the right atrium (RA) and diastolic collapse of the right ventricle. Tamponade was diagnosed and urgent pericardiocentesis was performed. View E-book for ultrasound clip or watch it at http://goo.gl/9IyuPR.

Tamponade is associated with (Figure 6.24a and b —clip):

- *Large-volume* pericardial effusion.
- Right atrial or ventricular *collapse during diastole*
- *Poorly collapsing inferior vena cava* during inspiration (which may even be dilated >20 mm in severe cases).

Tamponade requires urgent treatment with pericardiocentesis, which must only be performed by appropriately trained medical staff in an adequately staffed and equipped environment.

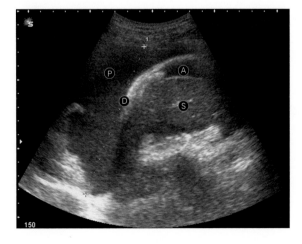

## ABDOMEN

The liver, spleen, and kidneys should be routinely located as part of a thoracic ultrasound scan, and physicians are encouraged to also examine the sonographic features of these organs. Given their proximity to the diaphragm, these structures are particularly useful in defining the inferior extent of the hemithorax when there is significant anatomical distortion, e.g., massively raised hemidiaphragm or consolidated lung mimicking the liver.

Recognition of commonly encountered abdominal pathology is essential if physicians are to avoid insertion of chest tubes into ascites, renal cysts, and other abdominal collections that may have similar sonographic characteristics to pleural effusions. Other abnormalities, such as hepatic metastases, are often visualized with ultrasound and can aid the diagnosis of malignancy.

*Ascites* may accompany a pleural effusion, particularly when transudative. The fluid is found abutting but inferior to the diaphragm, surrounding liver, or spleen and is frequently anechoic or hypoechoic (Figures 6.25, 6.26—clip, and 6.27—clip), although it may be septated.

**Figure 6.25** Ascites (A) adjacent to diaphragm (D), spleen (S), and a large echogenic pleural effusion (P).

CHAPTER 6

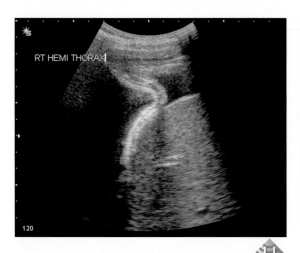

**Figure 6.26** Ascites adjacent to liver, diaphragm, and pleural effusion. Note the abnormal diaphragmatic movement. View E-book for ultrasound clip or watch it at http://goo.gl/EcaaWa.

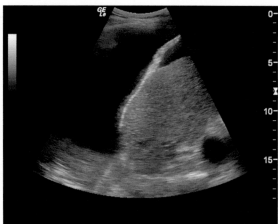

**Figure 6.27** Large pleural effusion and ascites in a patient with hepatic hydrothorax. Abnormal diaphragmatic movement again seen. View E-book for ultrasound clip or watch it at http://goo.gl/UK09a6.

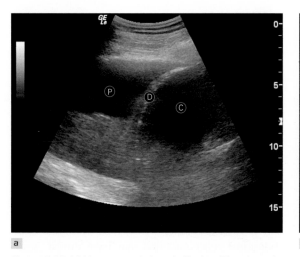

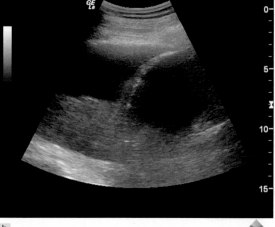

a

b

**Figure 6.28** (a) Nonseptated pleural effusion (P) and renal cyst (C) abutting the diaphragm (D), mimicking a septated effusion. (b) Nonseptated pleural effusion and renal cyst abutting a poorly moving diaphragm, mimicking a septated effusion. View E-book for ultrasound clip or watch it at http://goo.gl/SBG07s.

*Renal cysts* are occasionally seen and are usually easily visualized arising from the kidneys. When numerous and of significant size (e.g., with adult polycystic kidney disease), their relationship to the kidneys may be less apparent and they can mimic a septated pleural space (Figures 6.28a and b—clip).

*Hepatic metastases* may be visualized, although frequently have nonspecific appearances requiring further investigation for diagnosis. Multiple lesions of tissue echogenicity and of varying sizes are, however, strongly suspicious for metastases. The echogenicity of metastases vary, and may be *hypo-*, *iso-*, or *hyperechoic*, with isoechoic metastases being particularly difficult to identify. Other features may be seen, such as cystic metastases (which may be difficult to distinguish from other lesions, such as simple cysts or hepatic abscesses), calcification, necrosis, and hemorrhage (Figures 6.29a and b—clip).

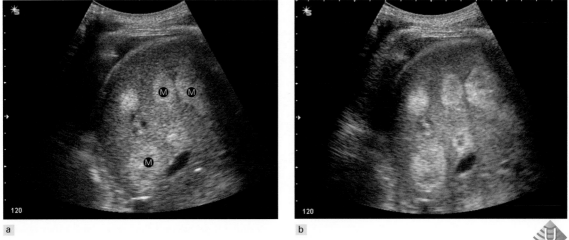

**Figure 6.29** (a) Multiple hyperechoic liver metastases (M) of varying sizes. (b) Multiple hyperechoic liver metastases of varying sizes. View E-book for ultrasound clip or watch it at http://goo.gl/tr6vUa.

## CHEST WALL

Optimal images of the chest wall are usually obtained using a high-frequency linear probe, enabling the visualization of abnormalities such as metastases and rib fractures.

Soft tissue and rib *metastases* may be evaluated and sampled under direct vision. In health, the only portion of rib visible is the anterior cortex—this appears as a *bright hyperechoic curved line* that casts a *posterior acoustic shadow*. Metastatic disease causing bony destruction can lead to *irregularity of the anterior cortex*, (partial) disappearance of the acoustic shadow, and the ability to image the infiltrated bone (which has a *hypoechoic, often heterogeneous*, structure). Soft tissue metastases have a similar hypoechoic rounded structure (Figure 6.30a and b—clip).

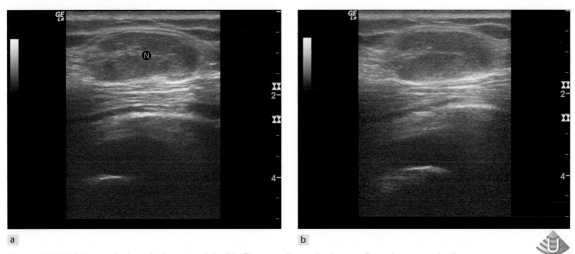

**Figure 6.30** (a) Hypoechoic soft tissue nodule (N). Fine-needle aspiration confirmed metastatic disease. (b) Hypoechoic soft tissue nodule. Fine-needle aspiration confirmed metastatic disease. View E-book for ultrasound clip or watch it at http://goo.gl/P50qn5.

*Rib fractures* are best detected by scanning longitudinally over ribs with a linear array transducer, and have the following features:

- A *gap*, *step*, or *frank dislocation* of the anterior rib cortex.
- *Reverberation echoes*, appearing as a "beam" below the edges of fractures, which are also known as "chimney" or "lighthouse" phenomena.
- Soft tissue edema or hematoma.
- *Accompanying findings* may also be seen, such as pleural fluid and parenchymal changes (due to lung contusion).

## CHEST TUBES AND INDWELLING PLEURAL CATHETERS

Ultrasound should be used to guide placement of chest tubes for pleural fluid, being associated with a significant reduction in risk of procedure-related complications[20] (see Chapter 9).

When inserted for pleural fluid (rather than pneumothorax), chest tubes and indwelling pleural catheters may be seen with ultrasound, and appear as *hyperechoic parallel lines* created by wave reflection at the edges of the catheter. If fluid filled, repetitive reflection between the two walls of the tube often creates further distal *artifactual parallel lines* (Figures 6.31 and 6.32—clip).

In addition to guiding insertion, bedside ultrasound may be used to ensure adequate drainage of a pleural effusion, enabling prompt removal of pleural catheters without the need for repeated chest radiography (Figure 6.33). The whole hemithorax should be scanned to accurately quantify any remaining fluid prior to tube removal, especially when fluid is loculated. When pleural fluid has failed to adequately resolve, and further therapy (such as surgery) is being considered, CT is a better technique to visualize the overall volume of residual fluid, pleural thickening, and other associated pathologies.

While it is relatively easy to confirm placement of a chest tube in pleural fluid, visualization of the entire course of the tube is difficult, and locating the tube tip may be particularly problematic. Detection of the tip may be facilitated by flushing the tube with sterile saline, creating an echogenic plume originating from the tube tip (caused by microbubbles within the saline).

Other tube features may also be visualized, including the side ports. Occasionally, indwelling catheters become occluded, and fibrinous material may be visualized within the tubing using ultrasound.

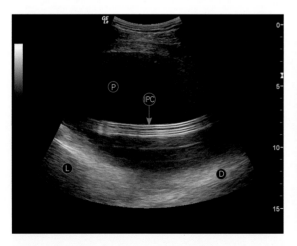

**Figure 6.31** Indwelling pleural catheter (IPC, arrow) seen within a large anechoic left pleural effusion (P). The diaphragm (D) and lung (L) are also visible.

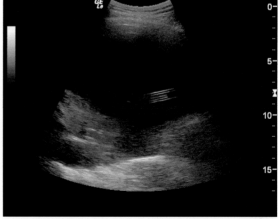

**Figure 6.32** Chest tube seen within a large pleural effusion. Atelectatic lung is also visible. View E-book for ultrasound clip or watch it at http://goo.gl/X8oNMU.

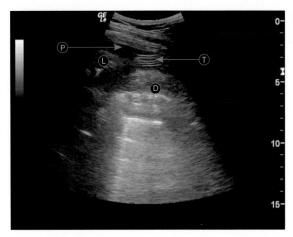

**Figure 6.33** Chest tube (T, arrow) within a small residual pleural effusion (P, arrow) at the costophrenic angle, adjacent to the diaphragm (D). The lung (L) had adequately reexpanded and the tube was removed after imaging the entire hemithorax.

 **TIPS FOR CLINICAL PRACTICE**

- Examine available cross-sectional imaging prior to ultrasound, to assist abnormality detection and image interpretation.
- Be aware of abdominal mimics of pleural disease—always find the liver, spleen, and kidneys to help define the inferior extent of the pleural space.
- Remember that consolidation may be difficult to distinguish from the liver.
- Routinely check for a pericardial effusion, particularly in the context of malignancy.
- Seek expert radiology guidance for any abdominal abnormalities detected.

# REFERENCES

1. Lichtenstein DA, Lascols N, Mezière G, Gepner A. Ultrasound diagnosis of alveolar consolidation in the critically ill. *Intensive Care Med* 2004; 30(2):276–281.

2. Gehmacher O, Mathis G, Kopf A, Scheier M. Ultrasound imaging of pneumonia. *Ultrasound Med Biol* 1995; 21(9):1119–1122.

3. Yang PC, Luh KT, Chang DB, Yu CJ, Kuo SH, Wu HD. Ultrasonographic evaluation of pulmonary consolidation. *Am Rev Respir Dis* 1992; 146(3):757–762.

4. Lichtenstein D, Mezière G, Seitz J. The dynamic air bronchogram. A lung ultrasound sign of alveolar consolidation ruling out atelectasis. *Chest* 2009; 135(6):1421–1425.

5. Yang PC, Luh KT, Lee YC, Chang DB, Yu CJ, Wu HD, et al. Lung abscesses: US examination and US-guided transthoracic aspiration. *Radiology* 1991; 180(1):171–175.

6. Yang PC, Luh KT, Wu HD, Chang DB, Lee LN, Kuo SH, et al. Lung tumors associated with obstructive pneumonitis: US studies. *Radiology* 1990; 174(3 Pt 1):717–720.

7. Yuan A, Chang DB, Yu CJ, Kuo SH, Luh KT, Yang PC. Color Doppler sonography of benign and malignant pulmonary masses. *AJR Am J Roentgenol* 1994; 163(3):545–549.

8. Yang PC. Ultrasound-guided transthoracic biopsy of peripheral lung, pleural, and chest-wall lesions. *J Thorac Imaging* 1997; 12(4):272–284.

9. Nakano N, Yasumitsu T, Kotake Y, Morino H, Ikezoe J. Preoperative histologic diagnosis of chest wall invasion by lung cancer using ultrasonically guided biopsy. *J Thoracic Cardiovasc Surg* 1994; 107(3):891–895.

10. Mathis G, Blank W, Reissig A, Lechleitner P, Reuss J, Schuler A, et al. Thoracic ultrasound for diagnosing pulmonary embolism: a prospective multicenter study of 352 patients. *Chest* 2005; 128(3):1531–1538.

11. Lichtenstein D, Mézière G, Biderman P, Gepner A, Barré O. The comet-tail artifact. An ultrasound sign of alveolar–interstitial syndrome. *Am J Respir Crit Care Med* 1997; 156(5):1640–1646.

12. Volpicelli G, Mussa A, Garofalo G, Cardinale L, Casoli G, Perotto F, et al. Bedside lung ultrasound in the assessment of alveolar-interstitial syndrome. *Am J Emerg Med* 2006; 24(6):689–696.

13. Copetti R, Soldati G, Copetti P. Chest sonography: a useful tool to differentiate acute cardiogenic pulmonary edema from acute respiratory distress syndrome. *Cardiovasc Ultrasound* 2008; 6:16.

14. Agricola E, Bove T, Oppizzi M, Marino G, Zangrillo A, Margonato A, et al. "Ultrasound comet-tail images": a marker of pulmonary edema: a comparative study with wedge pressure and extravascular lung water. *Chest* 2005; 127(5):1690–1695.

CHAPTER 6

15. Lichtenstein DA, Mezière GA, Lagoueyte J-F, Biderman P, Goldstein I, Gepner A. A-lines and B-lines: lung ultrasound as a bedside tool for predicting pulmonary artery occlusion pressure in the critically ill. *Chest* 2009; 136(4):1014–1020.

16. Lichtenstein D, Mézière G. A lung ultrasound sign allowing bedside distinction between pulmonary edema and COPD: the comet-tail artifact. *Intensive Care Med* 1998; 24(12):1331–1334.

17. Gerscovich EO, Cronan M, McGahan JP, Jain K, Jones CD, McDonald C. Ultrasonographic evaluation of diaphragmatic motion. *J Ultrasound Med* 2001; 20(6):597–604.

18. Gottesman E, McCool FD. Ultrasound evaluation of the paralyzed diaphragm. *Am J Respir Crit Care Med* 1997; 155(5):1570–1574.

19. Mandavia DP, Hoffner RJ, Mahaney K, Henderson SO. Bedside echocardiography by emergency physicians. *Ann Emerg Med* 2001; 38(4):377–382.

20. Wrightson JM, Fysh E, Maskell NA, Lee YC. Risk reduction in pleural procedures: sonography, simulation and supervision. *Curr Opin Pulm Med* 2010; 16(4):340–350.

CHAPTER 6

---

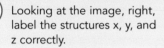

**MCQ 1**

**Q** Looking at the image, right, label the structures x, y, and z correctly.

a. x = aerated lung,
   y = pleural effusion,
   z = diaphragm.

b. x = aerated lung,
   y = pleural effusion,
   z = spleen.

c. x = consolidated lung,
   y = pleural effusion,
   z = diaphragm.

d. x = aerated lung,
   y = spleen,
   z = splenic hilum.

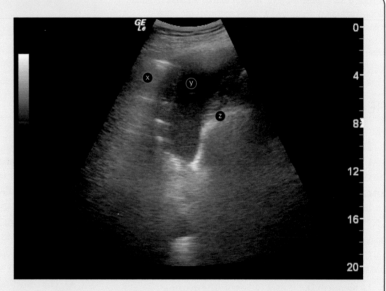

---

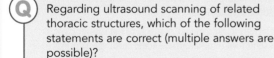

**MCQ 2**

**Q** Regarding ultrasound scanning of related thoracic structures, which of the following statements are correct (multiple answers are possible)?

a. The liver, spleen and kidneys should be routinely located as part of a thoracic ultrasound scan.

b. Features below the diaphragm on ultrasound can assist in the diagnosis of thoracic pathology.

c. Identification of a pericardial effusion on thoracic ultrasound removes the need for formal echocardiography.

d. The full dome-shaped diaphragm is clearly visualised in health, due to overlying aerated lung.

## MCQ 3

**Q** Looking at the image, right, label the structures w, x, y, and z correctly.

**a.** w = septations, x = heart, y = atelectatic lung, z = diaphragm.

**b.** w = pleural catheter within effusion, x = heart, y = atelectatic lung, z = diaphragm.

**c.** w = pleural catheter within renal cyst, x = heart, y = atelectatic lung, z = diaphragm.

**d.** w = pleural catheter within effusion, x = aorta, y = atelectatic lung, z = heart.

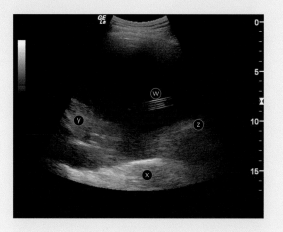

## ANSWERS

**1.** d

See the ultrasound clip, right, which confirms the vascular flow within the spleen. The spleen can be misinterpreted as an effusion in some circumstances. Drainage of this "pleural effusion" would have resulted in splenic trauma. Always be certain of where the diaphragm, spleen/liver, and kidney are. Color Doppler can be helpful.

**2.** a, b

The upper abdominal organs should be located at every scan to ensure correct anatomical location and orientation. Features below the diaphragm, such as ascites or liver metastases, can help point towards a diagnosis above the diaphragm, particularly in the case of pleural effusion. Normal aerated lung obscures the diaphragm in health, which may be better visualised (but still only partially) via the liver or spleen.

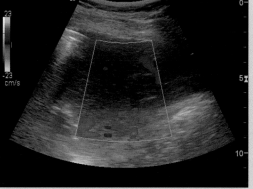

View E-book for ultrasound clip or watch it at http://goo.gl/98tkvl.

**3.** b

This indwelling pleural catheter was well located in a large free-flowing pleural effusion. The diaphragm was inverted, resulting in an abnormally obtuse angle between it and the mediastinum.

CHAPTER 6

# Pneumothorax

Sam Phillips and James Rippey

## INTRODUCTION

Pneumothorax is a common disorder in the critically ill, the trauma patient, and after iatrogenic procedures, and can be life threatening, requiring expeditious diagnosis and treatment.[1] Bedside radiography misses a high percentage of cases[2–6] and may underestimate the real volume involved. This is especially true with supine x-rays, which are notoriously inaccurate when looking for pneumothoraces, with sensitivities in blunt trauma of between 28 and 75%.[7] This is because free air layering anteriorly is projected over normal lung posteriorly and is difficult to see. Even tension pneumothoraces can be radio-occult,[8] and CT cannot be routinely used for this indication. Overuse of CT scanning can also lead to excessive irradiation of the patient, increased costs, and can subject patients to potential risks with medical transport.

Bedside ultrasound provides a noninvasive means to quickly assess for a pneumothorax as well as other life-threatening lung disorders with a sensitivity that may be an improvement on the current gold standard.[9]

Lung ultrasound was classically thought to be of limited use, since air is an impenetrable medium; however, it is the use of ultrasound artifacts that enables detection of a pneumothorax with the presence of several cardinal signs. These include absence of lung sliding, absence of comet tails and B lines, presence of a distinct A line, absence of a lung pulse, and visualization of a lung point. These important artifacts and their generation are explained below, as well as some of the common pitfalls (mimics) of these findings.

## TECHNIQUE

The patient is placed in the supine position and an ultrasound transducer is orientated in a longitudinal direction. Use of varying transducer types has been advocated by different authors. Some feel the coarse, more obvious artifact generation by a low-frequency probe (such as a phased-array echo probe) is best, while others feel the more precise definition offered by a higher-frequency probe (linear array) is better. The authors favor the standard curvilinear abdominal probe that utilizes the intermediate-frequency range.

The long axis of the probe should be aligned parallel to the long axis of the patient's body (vertical/longitudinal plane), initially viewing the anterior chest wall with the transducer placed over the third to fourth intercostal space and then moving inferiorly to the costo-diaphragmatic border. (Figures 7.1a and b—video). The transducer can then be moved laterally, to the right and left anterior axillary line in the third to fifth intercostal space, which is where the respiratory expansion of the lung is greater (and thus the amount of lung sliding increases).

7

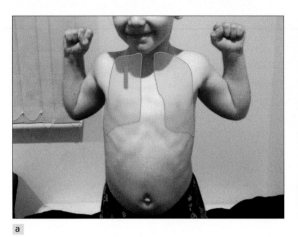

a   b

**Figure 7.1** (a) Ultrasound technique demonstrating the anterior approach with probe in the mid-clavicular line, third intercostal space (orange bar) with the patient supine or at 45°. Usually best for viewing a pneumothorax, as this is the most apical point of the thoracic cavity. (b) Ultrasound technique demonstrating the anterior, axillary, and posterior approach when searching for a pneumothorax. View E-book for video clip or watch it at http://goo.gl/6c4fhm.

## ULTRASONOGRAPHIC FEATURES OF A PNEUMOTHORAX

There are four important signs to assess for the presence of a pneumothorax.

### Sign 1: Absence of lung sliding

Pneumothorax should be sought first with an anterior examination approach, as 98% of significant cases are anterior in supine patients.[10]

The presence of lung sliding allows pneumothorax to be quickly and confidently discounted as a diagnosis since the negative predictive value of lung sliding is 100%.[11] It should be conceded that visualizing lung sliding in a single view means the two pleural surfaces are in contact at that point only. Pneumothorax may be present elsewhere in the thoracic cavity, and a thorough assessment of the entire thoracic cavity is required before concluding that there is no pneumothorax present.

The sliding lung sign is present when the visceral and parietal pleura are in contact, and move relative to one another during the respiratory cycle. When air separates the two pleural layers as in a pneumothorax, the movement disappears (Figures 7.2 and 7.3—videos). The free air deep to the parietal pleural completely excludes visualization of the visceral pleura and its movement.

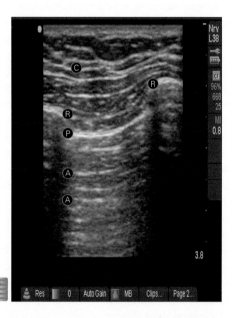

**Figure 7.2** Video demonstrating both normal lung and a pneumothorax showing loss of lung sliding, loss of lung pulse, loss of comet tails, loss of B lines, and dominant A lines (A). C = chest wall, R = rib, P = parietal pleura. View E-book for video clip or watch it at http://goo.gl/TKiiOS.

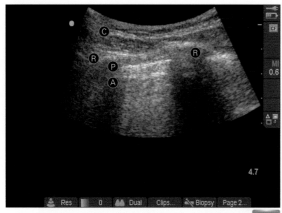

The visceral pleura is very slightly irregular, so rather than directly reflecting ultrasound back to the transducer, it is scattered in different directions, creating the appearance of an uneven surface that can be seen to slide up and down with normal respiration. In normal lung, occasional tiny pockets of interstitial fluid cause weak and fading short path reverberation artifacts known as comet tails, and these are projected deep to the pleural surface. These too can be seen to slide (unless there are adhesions or lack of lung movement), and these artifacts often make the sliding more apparent.

**Figure 7.3** Video demonstrating normal ventilating lung and a pneumothorax using curvilinear probe. Note the absence of lung sliding, loss of lung pulse, loss of comet tails, and B lines, and the presence of A lines. C = chest wall, R = ribs, P = parietal pleura, A = A lines. View E-book for video clip or watch it at http://goo.gl/7d2xXa.

There are three ways to assess the presence of lung sliding using ultrasound:

- The lung slide can be directly observed in real-time motion using two-dimensional ultrasonography, and images can be saved as video.
- Power Doppler can be used to highlight the motion of the pleura.
- M mode can be used to demonstrate lung sliding on a static image. When using M mode for this technique, follow a line that includes subcutaneous tissue, chest wall muscle, pleura, and lung. In a normal lung, the image obtained using M mode should demonstrate smooth lines superficially (because the chest wall shouldn't move with respiration in this view). Deep to the pleura, the sliding lung and very slightly irregular visceral pleural surface will produce enough motion artifact to create a rougher, grainier image producing the characteristic "waves on a beach" or "seashore" sign (Figures 7.4a and b—video).

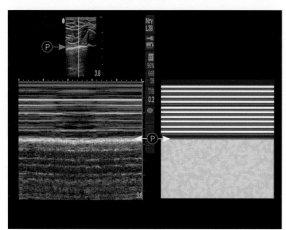

a

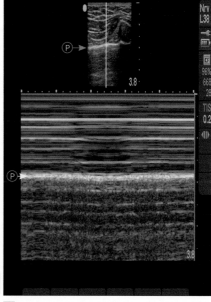

b

**Figure 7.4** (a) Normal lung ultrasound using M mode, demonstrating the "waves on a beach" or "seashore" sign. P = parietal pleura. (b) Video demonstration of (a). P = parietal pleura. View E-book for video clip or watch it at http://goo.gl/ZXGD0G.

**Figure 7.5** (a) Pneumothorax shown using M mode, giving the characteristic "waves" or "barcode" sign. P = parietal pleura. (b) Video demonstration of (a). P = parietal pleura. View E-book for video clip or watch it at http://goo.gl/asRTzz.

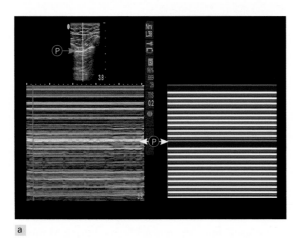

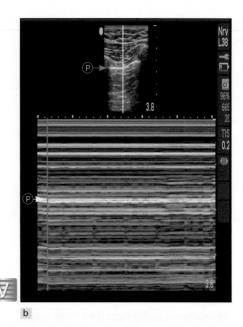

a

b

In the case of a pneumothorax, no motion will be visible in the chest wall or lung. The very smooth and flat parietal pleural surface, with free air below it, acts as a reflective surface. The resultant reverberation artifact creates further motionless horizontal lines, replicating those in the tissue superficial to the pleural surface, below it. This gives a characteristic "barcode" or "stratosphere" appearance (Figures 7.5a and b—video).

## Sign 2: Presence of A lines

A lines are repetitive horizontal echoic lines that arise from the pleural line at regular intervals (skin–pleural line distance) and are due to reverberations that occur due to the high acoustic impedance between the pleura and subpleural air, which completely reflects the ultrasound beam. An exclusive A line with no comet tails or B lines visible, even with extensive scanning, is called the A-line sign (Figure 7.6—video). The A-line sign is 100% sensitive for the diagnosis of a complete pneumothorax; however, it has a specificity of only 60%.[12] It is important to realize that although A lines may be visible to a depth of 10 cm or more, this does not mean the pneumothorax extends to this depth. A lines are generated through reverberation artifact at the pleural line, and so give no estimation of depth beyond this point.

The A-line sign and absent lung sliding when combined have a sensitivity and a negative predictive value of 100% and a specificity of 96.5%.[12]

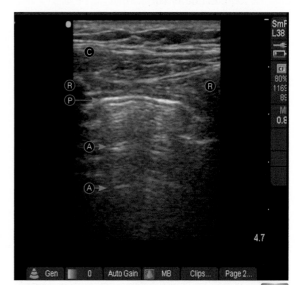

**Figure 7.6** Pneumothorax video demonstrating the A-line sign, with absence of comet tails or B lines, and multiple A lines. Visualization of chest wall (C), ribs (R), parietal pleura (P), and A lines (A) using linear probe. View E-book for video clip or watch it at http://goo.gl/PJGPoq.

## Sign 3: Lung pulse

This is the presence of a vertical movement of the pleural line synchronous to the cardiac rhythm and can be seen in the absence of lung sliding. It is caused by the transmission of the heartbeat through a motionless nonventilating lung. This lack of ventilation may be due to collapse/consolidation, or to apnea subsequent to pharmacological paralysis or simply by breath holding in the absence of disease.[13,14] This sign is very useful to differentiate a pneumothorax from other conditions characterized by absent lung sliding. In a study on patients with cardiac activity but absent lung sliding due to massive atelectasis and main stem intubation, lung pulse was a common finding, which allowed diagnosis with 93% sensitivity.[13] A pneumothorax, however, is characterized by both the absence of lung sliding and lung pulse, because the intrapleural air layer does not allow transmission of any movement of the parietal pleura. So the visualization of a lung pulse rules out a pneumothorax.[15]

## Sign 4: The lung point

The lung point is a highly specific sign that is seen only with a pneumothorax. It assumes that the absence of lung sliding and the presence of an A line have already been identified. The probe then needs to be gradually moved laterally until visualization of either lung

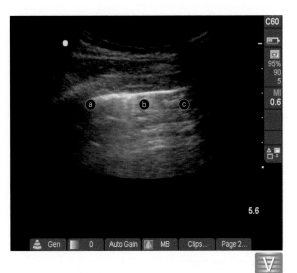

**Figure 7.7** Demonstration of a pneumothorax showing the lung point, where a = normal ventilating lung, b = contact or lung point, and c = pneumothorax. View E-book for video clip or watch it at http://goo.gl/oCPC5n.

sliding with or without comet tails and B lines during inspiration can be recorded. Here the lung is now in contact with the chest wall and represents the border of the pneumothorax. The lung point can be visualized in B mode and M mode (Figures 7.7—video and 7.8a and b—video. The specificity of the lung point is 100%

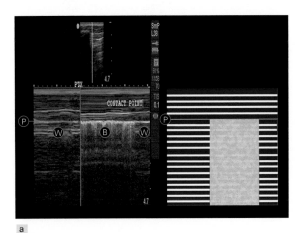

a

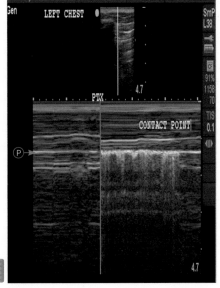

b

**Figure 7.8** (a) Image demonstrating the contact or lung point using M mode, where W = "barcode/wave" appearance of a pneumothorax, followed by the "beach" appearance (B) of normal ventilating lung, before a further wave appearance after this. (P) = parietal pleura. (b) Video demonstrating the contact or lung point using M mode. P = parietal pleura. View E-book for video clip or watch it at http://goo.gl/7RLvtC.

with an overall sensitivity of 66%, which decreases in the case of major pneumothorax with complete lung retraction.[14]

The lung point confirms that the absence of lung sliding is real and is not due to technical faults. The lung point also provides an indication of the pneumothorax volume and allows monitoring of the state of a pneumothorax. An anterior lung point indicates a moderate pneumothorax, whereas a very posterior or absent lung point suggests a large pneumothorax. In one study, a lateral lung point was correlated with a 90% need for drainage, versus 8% with the presence of an anterior lung point.[16] It is important to appreciate, however, that no treatment guidelines currently advocate the use of ultrasound to determine pneumothorax management.

## COMMON ULTRASONOGRAPHIC MIMICS OF A PNEUMOTHORAX

There are a number of conditions that may mimic a pneumothorax with the absence of lung sliding. This is especially true in the critically unwell, with the absence of lung sliding having a positive predictive value of only 56%.[17] Certain conditions that lead to this are jet or high-frequency ventilation (with low tidal volumes), massive atelectasis (including one lung intubation), emphysema and bullae (Figure 7.9—video), acute pleural inflammation with adherence, chronic adhesion secondary to previous chemical or surgical pleurodesis, and severe fibrosis.

There are also three important mimics of the lung point that should be recognized. The lung interface with the heart in the left chest can be mistaken for a lung point, and so can the inferior edge of the lung at the diaphragm. The first two mimics should be quickly detected by a close look at the surrounding anatomy. The third occurs at the edge of a large bulla where relatively normal lung abuts a collection of air within the bulla and may mislead the unwary sonographer.

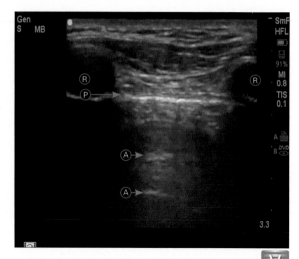

**Figure 7.9** Video showing an emphysematous bulla with the same sonographic features as a pneumothorax, with loss of lung sliding, comet tails, and B lines, and accentuation of A lines. R = ribs, P = parietal pleura, A = A lines. View E-book for video clip or watch it at http://goo.gl/c26hjj.

Subcutaneous emphysema may also hinder the diagnosis of a pneumothorax, as it may lead to a false view of pleural motion and vertical artifacts similar to B lines called "E lines". The important differences with E lines, however, are that these vertical lines originate above the pleural line and do not slide with ventilation (Figure 7.10a and b—video). This compares with B lines that arise from the pleural line, slide with ventilation, and can exclude a pneumothorax if present.

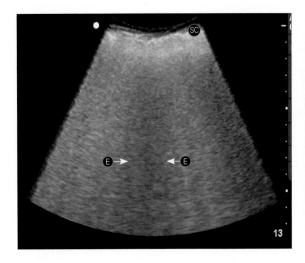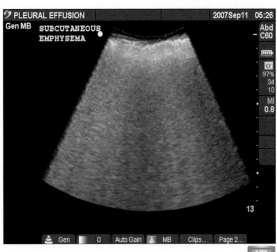

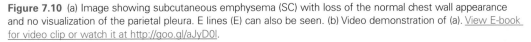

**Figure 7.10** (a) Image showing subcutaneous emphysema (SC) with loss of the normal chest wall appearance and no visualization of the parietal pleura. E lines (E) can also be seen. (b) Video demonstration of (a). View E-book for video clip or watch it at http://goo.gl/aJyD0l.

## CONCLUSION

Ultrasound is a very useful tool in the immediate bedside diagnosis of pneumothorax, but it is not without potential pitfalls. The clinician must consider the possible presence of underlying lung disease, the level of clinical suspicion (pretest probability), and must integrate this knowledge with the results of the investigation to reach a final considered conclusion.

If ultrasound findings are typical for pneumothorax in a young patient, with normal lungs, presenting after chest trauma, then the diagnosis is almost certainly pneumothorax. On the other hand, if a patient with known emphysematous bullae and previous pleurodesis presents with increasing shortness of breath, findings suggestive of pneumothorax would be very difficult to differentiate from large nonsliding subpleural bullae.

### TIPS FOR CLINICAL PRACTICE

- Set your depth and focus to look at the parietal pleural surface optimally. Anything behind this point is just artifact.

- Put the probe where you would expect to see free air and hold the probe very still, watching for lung sliding. If there is no sliding, slowly move the probe downward looking for a contact or lung point. M mode and power Doppler will not clarify a situation that is not clear already.

- It is essential to marry your ultrasound findings with your clinical suspicion. Conditions causing hypoventilation and loss of normal lung parenchyma (such as bullous emphysema) can mimic pneumothorax.

- Practice.

CHAPTER 7

# REFERENCES

1. Lichtenstein D, Loubière Y. Lung ultrasonography in pulmonary embolism [Letter]. *Chest* 2003; 123:2154.

2. Tocino IM, Miller MH, Fairfax WR. Distribution of pneumothorax in the supine and semi-recumbent critically ill adult. *AJR Am J Roentgenol* 1985; 144:901–5.

3. Steier M, Ching N, Roberts EB, et al. Pneumothorax complicating ventilatory support. *J Thorac Cardiovasc Surg* 1974; 67:17–23.

4. Hill SL, Edmisten T, Holtzman G, et al. The occult pneumothorax: an increasing diagnostic entity in trauma. *Am Surg* 1999; 65:254–58.

5. Kurdziel JC, Dondelinger RF, Hemmer M. Radiological management of blunt polytrauma with CT and angiography: an integrated approach. *Ann Radiol* 1987;30:121–24.

6. McGonigal MD, Schwab CW, Kauder DR, et al. Supplemented emergent chest CT in the management of blunt torso trauma. *J Trauma* 1990; 30:1431–35.

7. Wilkerson RG, Stone MB. Sensitivity of bedside ultrasound and supine anteroposterior chest radiographs for the identification of pneumothorax after blunt trauma. *Acad Emerg Med* 2010; 17(1):11.

8. Gobien RP, Reines HD, Schabel SI. Localized tension pneumothorax: unrecognized form of barotrauma in ARDS. *Radiology* 1982; 142:15–19.

9. Rowan KR, Kirkpatrick AW, Liu D, et al. Traumatic pneumothorax detection with US: correlation with chest radiography and CT—initial experience. *Radiology* 2002; 225(1):210–14.

10. Lichtenstein D, Holzapfel L, Frija J. Cutaneous projection of pneumothorax and impact on the ultrasound diagnosis. *Réan Urg* 2000; 9(Suppl 2):138s.

11. Lichtenstein DA, Menu Y. A bedside ultrasound sign ruling out pneumothorax in the critically ill. Lung sliding. *Chest* 1995; 108:1345–48.

12. Lichtenstein D, Mezière G, Biderman P, et al. The comet-tail artifact: an ultrasound sign ruling out pneumothorax. *Intensive Care Med* 1999; 25:383–88.

13. Lichtenstein DA, Lascols N, Prin S, Mezière G. The lung pulse: an early ultrasound sign of complete atelectasis. *Intensive Care Med* 2003; 29:2187–92.

14. Chun R, Kirkpatrick AW, Sirois M, Sargasyn AE, Melton S, Hamilton DR, Dulchavsky S. Where's the tube? Evaluation of hand-held ultrasound in confirming endotracheal tube placement. *Prehosp Disast Med* 2004; 19:366–69.

15. Volpicelli G. Sonographic diagnosis of pneumothorax. *Intensive Care Med* 2011; 37:224–32.

16. Lichtenstein DA, Mezière G, Lascols N, et al. Ultrasound diagnosis of occult pneumothorax. *Crit Care Med* 2005; 33:1231–38.

17. Lichtenstein D, Mezière G, Biderman P, et al. The "lung point": an ultrasound sign specific to pneumothorax. *Intensive Care Med* 2000; 26:1434–40.

## MCQ 1

**Q** A young patient with previously normal lungs was involved in a motor vehicle accident and presents with some chest pain. This ultrasound clip is taken on the side of pain, in the third intercostal space in the mid-clavicular line. Pick the most correct answer.

**a.** This ultrasound excludes the presence of pneumothorax.

**b.** This ultrasound demonstrates lung sliding and comet-tail artifact.

**c.** This ultrasound shows prominent A lines.

**d.** A lung or contact point is seen in this clip.

**e.** In this case, using power Doppler would help clarify findings.

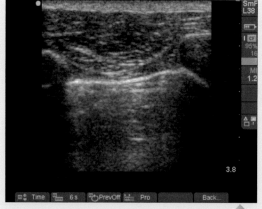

View E-book for ultrasound clip or watch it at http://goo.gl/rltmgK.

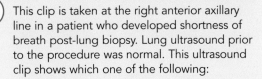

## MCQ 2

This clip is taken at the right anterior axillary line in a patient who developed shortness of breath post-lung biopsy. Lung ultrasound prior to the procedure was normal. This ultrasound clip shows which one of the following:

a. Normal lung?

b. A moderate-sized hemothorax?

c. Contact or lung point confirming the presence of pneumothorax?

d. Pulmonary edema?

e. Surgical/subcutaneous emphysema?

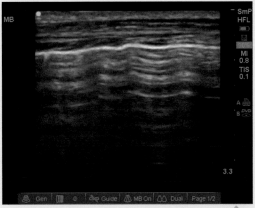

View E-book for ultrasound clip or watch it at http://goo.gl/Hkj97T.

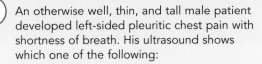

## MCQ 3

An otherwise well, thin, and tall male patient developed left-sided pleuritic chest pain with shortness of breath. His ultrasound shows which one of the following:

a. Z lines typical of surgical emphysema.

b. An M-mode demonstration of pneumothorax.

c. Normal ventilating lung.

d. Lung-pulse sign.

e. Pneumothorax.

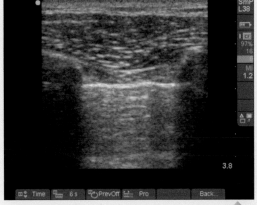

View E-book for ultrasound clip or watch it at http://goo.gl/idFHxV.

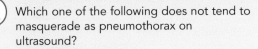

## MCQ 4

Which one of the following does not tend to masquerade as pneumothorax on ultrasound?

a. Pleural effusion.

b. Nonventilating lung (such as in rightmain stem intubation).

c. Lung bullae.

d. Surgical or subcutaneous emphysema.

e. Pleurodesis.

CHAPTER 7

**ANSWERS**

**1.** b

This clip shows normal lung sliding with comet-tail artifact. This means the visceral and parietal pleura are sliding against each other and exclude the presence of free air between the pleural surfaces—at that point only. In a supine patient with otherwise normal lungs, free air would be expected to collect at the site being examined. However, tiny pneumothoraces, or those with pleural adhesions and loculated pneumothoraces, cannot be excluded completely.

**2.** c

The patient has a moderate-sized pneumo-thorax with the two pleural surfaces meeting in the right anterior axillary line. On the left of the image normal lung sliding and comet-tail artifacts are seen. On the right pneumothorax is seen. This point of contact is known as the lung or contact point.

**3.** e

This is a demonstration of a pneumothorax with loss of lung sliding, comet tails, and B lines, and prominent A lines. There is no surgical emphysema, which tends to hide the chest wall. It is not a still M-mode image. There is no lung pulse (transmitted mediastinal movement seen in nonventilating but otherwise normal lungs).

**4.** a

Pleural fluid tends to be black deep to the parietal pleural surface, with collapsed lung seen deep to it. Nonventilating lung and pleurodesis lead to loss of lung sliding, and surgical emphysema hides lung movement deep to it. Lung bullae can emulate pneumothoraces extremely well (see Chapter 7).

# Artifacts, Pitfalls, and Limitations

Nicola Smith and James Entwisle

## INTRODUCTION

The quality of the information obtained from an ultrasound scan is determined by the skill and knowledge of the user, and the ability of the user to recognize and minimize artifacts. This chapter will discuss the most common artifacts encountered in ultrasound of the chest and techniques to avoid these. It should be noted, however, that this is a skill best acquired in real time at the bedside from those experienced in pleural ultrasound.

Imaging artifacts can cause misdiagnosis by suggesting the presence of structures that are not present, or by obscuring important structures or pathology. A good example is reverberation artifact, which may give the false impression of adhesions or solid structures in a pleural effusion. If this is not recognized as artifact, it may result in the misdiagnosis of a simple pleural effusion as loculated, so influencing subsequent management decisions. It is essential for clinicians performing bedside pleural ultrasound to have an understanding of common artifacts, how they arise, how to recognize them, and to learn techniques to minimize their effect. Failure to do so may result in clinically significant errors in interpretation. This chapter will also discuss limitations to bedside pleural ultrasound, and pitfalls or errors that are commonly encountered by the novice.

## COMMON ARTIFACTS IN PLEURAL ULTRASOUND

### Reverberation artifact

Reverberation artifact occurs when the sound waves produced by the transducer are reflected repeatedly back and forth between the transducer and the interface. This causes multiple reflections, and multiple representations of the same interface in the image (see Chapters 2 and 4 for image examples).

Reverberation artifact may be seen within pleural effusions, appearing as multiple white lines in the fluid, usually superficially near the parietal pleura. It is regularly spaced because the time for each additional echo is a multiple of the time of return of the first echo. Reverberation artifact can give the false impression of septations in pleural fluid. It can be identified by the regularity of the lines, and the way in which the reflected echoes move with the probe. Reducing the overall gain can reduce reverberation artifact, as the artifactual echoes are weaker than the true ones, so as the overall image darkens, the artifact is minimized.

Comet-tail artifact is another type of reverberation artifact seen in normal lung. It appears as vertically oriented lines and occurs at the pleura–lung interface where there is a large change in acoustic impedance between the fluid-rich interlobular septae and the surrounding air-filled lung. Comet-tail artifact is lost when a pneumothorax is present (see Chapter 7), and the appearance of comet tails may be increased in the presence of pulmonary edema (see Figure 10.17, page 129).

### Refraction

When a sound beam moves through tissues with differing speeds of sound, i.e., from fluid to soft tissue, it is deviated in its path and does not move in a straight plane. This is called refraction.

Because ultrasound systems operate on the assumption that ultrasound beams move in a straight line, and that the speed of sound is constant in all body tissues (assumed as 1540 m/s), refraction can result in misregistration of echoes on the display. If the refraction

8

artifact is not identified, errors can be made in the precise location of anatomical structures, and structures may appear in the image that actually lie outside the area the operator assumes is being examined. As with most artifacts, the refraction artifact will move with the probe, so altering the probe position or scanning in a different plane and observing the effect on the artifact should help to identify the problem.

## Side-lobe artifact

Side-lobe artifact also arises from the assumption of the ultrasound operating system that ultrasound beams move in a straight line. However, the actual ultrasound beam has several side lobes that lie outside the main beam. These side lobes are reflected off tissue interfaces, and the resulting echoes transmitted to the transducer. The returning echoes are assumed by the machine to come from the central beam and are placed in the middle of the screen. This can be commonly seen when scanning the thorax and can cause the impression of solid structures or debris in pleural fluid (see Figure 2.13, page 17).

## Mirror-image artifact

Mirror-image artifact occurs where there is a strong specular reflector, which acts as a mirror, causing structures to be displayed twice, with one image being a mirror image of the other. This is most commonly seen in pleural ultrasound at the interface between the diaphragm and the lung, as the diaphragm is a very strong reflector. The liver or spleen can be falsely seen on both sides on the diaphragm (see Figure 4.28, page 56).

## Shadowing

Posterior acoustic shadowing is common in pleural ultrasound and can result in important pathology being obscured. This type of shadowing occurs where there is a large impedance mismatch between tissue interfaces resulting in a large percentage of sound being reflected. In pleural ultrasound the main difficulty with obscured images occurs with shadowing from ribs or the scapulae. At the interface between bone and soft tissue a large proportion of the sound wave is reflected. This causes partial or complete loss of information deep to the bony structure and is represented on the image as a black area behind the white interface of the rib or scapula. Thus, the operator cannot "see" beyond to the structures below (Figure 8.1). Bony shadowing is easily identified and can be avoided by altering the angle of the probe or changing the transducer to fit easily between the patient's ribs, or asking the patient to elevate his or her arm above his or her head.

## Operator-produced artifacts

A common mistake made by the beginner is a lack of contact between the probe and the chest wall. Liberal use of gel is encouraged, as is pressing firmly enough so that the maximum surface of the probe is in contact with the skin.

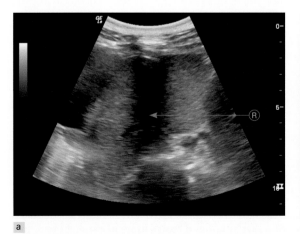
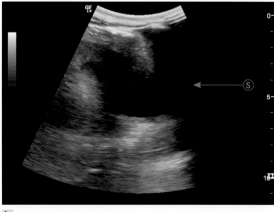

**Figure 8.1** Examples of posterior shadowing (R and S) caused by rib in (a) and the scapula in (b). At the interface between bone and soft tissue, the sound wave is reflected, causing loss of information deep to the bone. Thus, the operator cannot see beyond the bone to the structures below.

CHAPTER 8

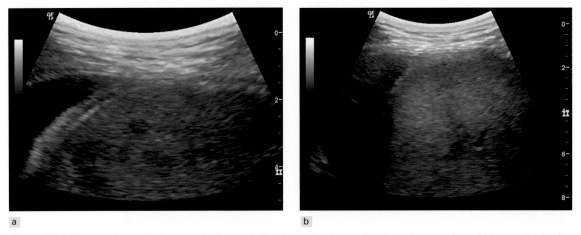

**Figure 8.2** (a) Image obtained when the diaphragm is first located, prior to alteration of any settings. (b) Image obtained from the same location after depth has been increased. Depth should be altered so that the interface between the pleural effusion at its maximum depth and the underlying compressed lung is seen.

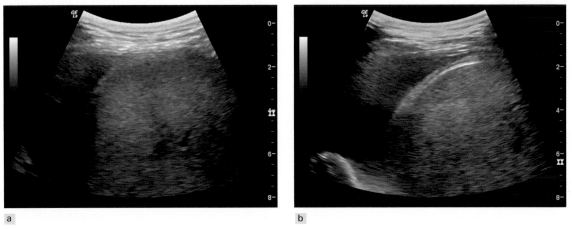

**Figures 8.3** (a) Before alteration of the focal zone. (b) The focal zone has been adjusted to 6 cm to focus on the interface between the pleural effusion at its maximum depth and the underlying compressed lung.

Further artifact is produced by inappropriate adjustment of the machine settings, in particular time-gain compensation (TGC) and gain. It is tempting when presented with a confusing image to turn up the gain in the hope that the image will become clearer; however, overuse will add to the noise of the image. Clinicians learning pleural ultrasound are advised to avoid the use of the gain and auto gain controls, and attempt to optimize the image by systematically adjusting the depth, focus, TGC, and frequency. With increasing skill and experience, the operator will learn to adjust the machine settings to display the best image, providing maximum information with minimum noise.

Depth should be selected so that the maximal depth is at the structure of most interest (often the diaphragm), or at the interface between the pleural effusion at its maximum depth and the underlying compressed lung (Figure 8.2). Lateral resolution should also be considered. If the lateral resolution is poor, two separate structures may appear as one image on the screen. The lateral resolution is best at the narrowest part of the ultrasound beam. Adjusting the focal zone to the area of most interest will focus the narrowest part of the beam on this area, hence improving lateral resolution (Figure 8.3).

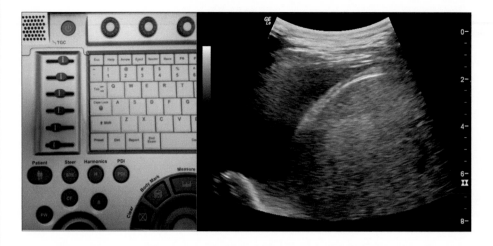

**Figure 8.4** The potentiometers should be moved together to stay in alignment.

The TGC can be adjusted to enhance weak echoes returning from deeper structures, but the potentiometers should be moved together to stay in alignment (Figures 8.4a, b). If one of the TGC controls is misaligned, a band of bright white or dark echoes may appear in the middle of the image (see Chapter 2 for image examples). TGC allows the operator to decide which part of the image needs to be enhanced. This contrasts with gain, which will amplify the whole of the received signal, affecting the whole image equally. Undue increases in gain may produce artifactual echoes in the fluid.

## TIPS FOR CLINICAL PRACTICE

The authors use the following approach when scanning the chest to minimize artifact and optimise the image obtained:

1. Locate the diaphragm.
2. Alter the depth so that the diaphragm is the deepest image on the screen, usually 12–15 cm.
3. Adjust the focal zone to the area of interest.
4. Adjust TGC if necessary.
5. Alter the frequency of the probe if necessary, especially if the patient has a large body habitus (lowering the frequency may aid image acquisition in this scenario).
6. Identify any possible artifacts on the image, i.e., reverberation, side-lobe artifact, etc.

7. If artifact is present alter the angulation of the probe, followed by scanning in both the horizontal and vertical plane in one position to observe the effect on the image. If artifact is present it will move with the probe. Similarly ask the patient to take some deep breaths and observe the movement with respiration.
8. If the image is still sub-optimal, change the position of the patient and scan again.
9. If looking at superficial structures, a linear high frequency probe can be used.
10. If there is difficulty identifying artifact, or interpreting the image obtained, stop the scan and organize for the patient to have a formal departmental scan by an ultrasonographer/radiologist.

CHAPTER 8

# COMMON PROBLEMS IN USER INTERPRETATION OF THE PLEURAL SPACE

For the novice there are several limitations commonly encountered in ultrasound of the chest. These can be divided into patient factors and pathological factors.

## Patient factors

Patient factors include body habitus, chest wall deformities, and patient cooperation. Obesity is an increasingly common barrier to obtaining good images of the pleural space. Excessive adipose tissue covering the chest wall can make visualization of deeper structure difficult due to increased absorption of the sound waves. This can usually be overcome by using a lower-frequency transducer to penetrate deeper, although this will also result in decreased resolution deeper in the field. Subtle abnormalities of the chest wall and parietal pleura may be obscured.

Chest wall deformities can also be problematic. In this situation attempting to angle the probe between the patient's ribs can usually overcome this difficulty. If this is not possible because of rib crowding, asking the patient to raise his or her arm above his or her head can expand the rib spaces, increasing the window between them and enabling better views. If the patient is unable to cooperate with the examination, by lying/sitting in the necessary position, changing position as required, etc., then an alternative mode of examination, such as computed tomography (CT), may be more useful.

## Pathological factors

Problems in interpretation related to the underlying pathology include the presence of air in the pleural space, subcutaneous emphysema, atelectatic lung, loculated fluid, and solid masses. The presence of air in the pleural space may be encountered in the patient with a malignant pleural effusion and "trapped lung," following any pleural procedure where air is introduced into the pleural space, or in the presence of a bronchopleural fistula. Where free air exists in the pleural space (pneumothorax), the normal lung sliding sign is lost (see Chapter 7). The free air–soft tissue interface reflects almost all sound waves, causing obscuration of deeper structures.

When both air and fluid are present in the pleural space, air fluid levels may be seen. The locules of air will produce bright linear interfaces with reverberation artifacts, which contrast with the dark anechoic fluid of the pleural effusion. This can produce confusing images for the novice (see Figure 5.13, page 65). If the chest x-ray has been examined prior to the ultrasound examination, and the air fluid levels identified, this can be correlated with the ultrasound images obtained, aiding in interpretation. A hydropneumothorax will produce a different image appearance, again one that can be difficult to interpret for the beginner (see Figure 5.19, page 68).

Subcutaneous emphysema, the presence of air in the subcutaneous tissues, will cause obscuration of deeper structures (see Figure 7.10b, page 97) and ultrasound should not be used in these patients. The presence of subcutaneous emphysema may indicate the presence of a pneumothorax, and chest x-ray or CT in this situation is likely to be a better choice of imaging modality.

Atelectatic lung is commonly seen when a large pleural effusion is present. This can occasionally be mistaken for a pleural mass. Atelectatic lung has a characteristic sonographic appearance, and should be easily differentiated from pleural pathology. Atelectatic lung appears as a wedge-shaped opacity, which "floats" through the pleural fluid in time with the patient's cardiac pulsation. Atelectatic lung is echogenic, and has sharp borders defined by visceral pleura (Figure 8.5).

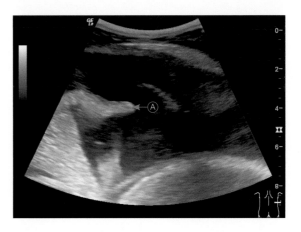

**Figure 8.5** Atelectatic lung (A) appears as a wedge-shaped opacity, which "floats" through the pleural fluid in time with the patient's cardiac pulsation. It is highly echogenic and has sharp borders defined by visceral pleura.

In contrast, pleural metastases or masses usually appear as nodular mid-echoic masses, which do not float as freely with respiration/cardiac pulsation, and can appear fixed to the pleura (Figures 8.6—clip and 8.7). Other sonographic signs of malignant pleural disease, such as pleural thickening, are usually present with pleural metastases and should be looked for to aid in differentiation.

Loculated pleural effusions can be easily missed on pleural ultrasound, especially if located in an anterior position. It is therefore important to scan the entirety of the hemithorax to ensure loculated pockets of fluid are not missed.

Echogenic complex pleural fluid, as seen with hemothorax and heavily septated effusion/empyema, may occasionally be difficult to differentiate from solid tissue in the pleural space (Figures 8.8a and b—clip). These two pathologies may also have similar sonographic appearances, and thoracentesis may be required to differentiate between the two. The appearance of blood on ultrasound depends on its age and whether it has begun to organize. Hemothorax can appear as a complex mass above the diaphragm.

Other large masses, such as a sarcoma, may be difficult to differentiate from an organized hematoma in a patient with an opacified hemithorax on chest x-ray. In this rare situation color Doppler can be used to distinguish between the two. A solid tumor (both primary and metastatic) will have a color Doppler signal as it has vascularity. An organized hematoma should have no Doppler signal.

> ### TIPS FOR CLINICAL PRACTICE
>
> - Always correlate the ultrasound appearances with a recent chest x-ray.
> - Echogenic fluid represents pus or hemothorax.
> - If the ultrasound and chest x-ray images do not correlate consider a repeat chest x-ray or CT scan.

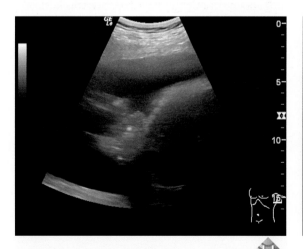

**Figure 8.6** Pleural metastasis. The nodular mid-echoic mass appears fixed to the pleura and does not float freely with respiration. View E-book for ultrasound clip or watch it at http://goo.gl/OplaRO.

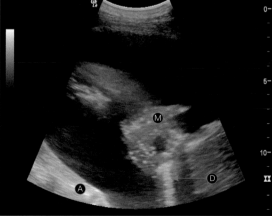

**Figure 8.7** Pleural metastasis (M) should be differentiated from atelectatic lung (A). D = diaphragmatic thickening.

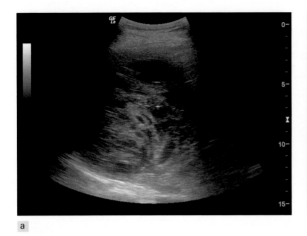
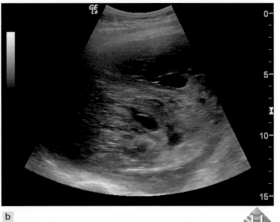

**Figure 8.8** (a) Ultrasound appearance of a malignant pleural effusion in a patient who had undergone two prior chest drain insertions. The appearance of a complex mass in the pleural fluid is suggestive of hemothorax. (b) Ultrasound clip of complex pleural space. View E-book for ultrasound clip or watch it at http://goo.gl/WdQkoS.

## Common errors during ultrasound-guided pleural procedures

Two of the most common errors made by the clinician inexperienced in bedside pleural ultrasound are a failure to adequately scan the entire chest and a failure to appreciate when it is unsafe to proceed with an invasive pleural procedure.

The former usually arises from a lack of time. One of the attractive features of bedside pleural ultrasound is the ability to quickly identify a pleural effusion to enable safe aspiration. The temptation is to simply place the transducer on the chest wall, confirm that fluid is present, and mark a spot for aspiration. This approach can lead to a failure to appreciate the extent of the effusion, and overlook important pathological features such as septations. This approach is also more likely to result in misinterpretation of artifact. An ultrasound examination of the chest wall should be undertaken in a systematic manner, scanning the entire chest wall. A "point and shoot" approach is best avoided.

Bedside pleural ultrasound has been shown to improve the safety of pleural procedures. This involves using the sonographic appearance to decide when it is safe to proceed with thoracentesis/chest drain insertion. The following ultrasound appearances should cause hesitation before proceeding with invasive procedures and prompt consideration of alternative methods of making the diagnosis:

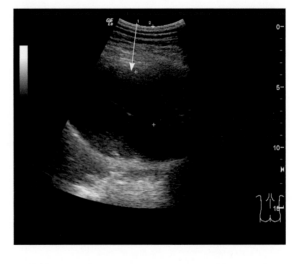

**Figure 8.9** If the distance from the skin to the pleural effusion (arrow) is greater than the length of the needle, aspiration is unlikely to be successful.

- The distance from the chest wall to the effusion is greater than the length of the needle to be used for aspiration (Figure 8.9).
- Excessive excursions of the diaphragm with respiration are present.

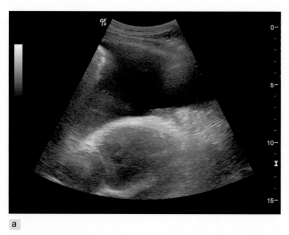

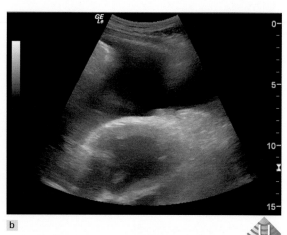

**Figure 8.10** (a) The left ventricle of the heart underneath a left pleural effusion. Visualization of the heart immediately below the effusion should prompt reevaluation of the safety of proceeding with pleural intervention. Ideally aspiration should be performed under direct ultrasound guidance. (b) Ultrasound clip of the same patient showing the pumping left ventricle of the heart underneath a left pleural effusion. View E–book for ultrasound clip or watch it at http://goo.gl/830rEZ.

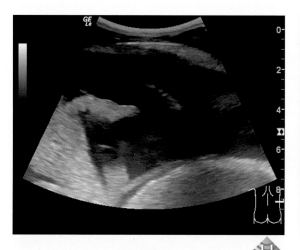

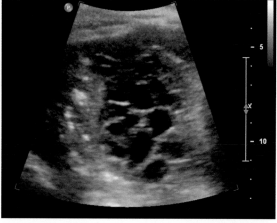

**Figure 8.11** Atelectatic lung floating freely in the pleural space very close to the line of intended needle insertion. View E-book for ultrasound clip or watch it at http://goo.gl/AS7zAv.

**Figure 8.12** A heavily loculated effusion. Simple chest tube drainage may not be successful in this scenario.

- The presence of a solid organ or major vessel adjacent to a small effusion, e.g., left ventricle of the heart (Figures 8.10a and b—video).
- Large amounts of atelectatic lung floating in the pleural fluid, which may be difficult to avoid when entering the pleural space (Figure 8.11).
- Access to the pleural effusion impeded by the scapula.

- A very medially located pleural effusion. Thoracentesis at this site posteriorly can increase the risk of laceration of the intercostal artery (see Chapters 4 and 9).
- A heavily loculated or septated pleural effusion where simple chest tube drainage may be less likely to be successful (Figure 8.12).

# FURTHER READING

*Introduction to ultrasound for respiratory physicians* (unpublished). Australian Institute of Ultrasound course notes. Gold Coast: Australian Institute of Ultrasound, 2010.

Koh D, Burke S, Davies N, Padley S. Transthoracic US of the chest: clinical uses and applications. *Radiographics* 2002: 22 e1.

Rumack C, Wilson S, Charboneau J, Johnson J. *Diagnostic ultrasound*, 3rd ed. Philadelphia: Elsevier Mosby, 2004: 3–33.

---

## MCQ 1

**Q** Which one of the following types of artifact is demonstrated in this image?

**a.** Posterior acoustic shadowing.

**b.** Posterior acoustic enhancement.

**c.** Mirror-image artifact.

**d.** Reverberation artifact.

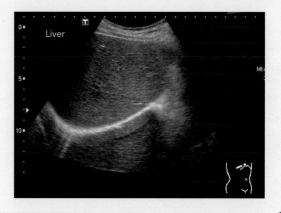

---

## MCQ 2

**Q** This image (a) has been optimized (b) by altering which one of the following?

**a.** Probe frequency.

**b.** Depth.

**c.** TGC (time-gain compensation).

**d.** Number of focal zones.

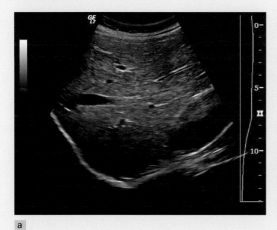

a

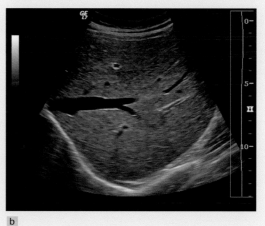

b

CHAPTER 8

**MCQ 3**

If an ultrasound image is sub-optimal, which of the following methods can help improve image acquisition? (multiple answers possible)

a. Changing the position of the patient.

b. Ensuring the gain is turned up high.

c. Altering the probe angulation and orientation.

d. Lowering the frequency of the probe when scanning a patient with a large body habitus.

**ANSWERS**

**1.** c

See Chapter 8 and Chapter 2 for artifact explanations and examples.

**2.** c

The probe frequency, depth, and number of focal zones (as illustrated by the small triangles to the right of the scale bar) are the same for both images. The spurious dark stripe across the liver in the first image is caused by an incorrectly set TGC. See Chapter 2 for details.

**3.** a, c, d

All of these manoeuvres may be helpful, except turning the gain up too high. This is a mistake often made by novice users; instead of improving image quality it will increase the noise of the image, thus making things less clear.

CHAPTER 8

# Real-Time Ultrasound-Guided Pleural Procedures

Christopher Gilbert and David Feller-Kopman

## INTRODUCTION

Advancements in technology over the last several years have allowed for the development of portable ultrasound units that can provide real-time, point-of-care assessment for a variety of diseases as well as guide diagnostic and therapeutic procedures. The use of ultrasound to guide pleural procedures requires a basic understanding of the physics and principles of ultrasonography, the knobology of the specific ultrasound unit being used, as well as skills in image acquisition and image interpretation. In addition to these skills, the operator must also be expert at performing the procedure without ultrasound guidance, and then develop the psychomotor coordination to perform the skills using ultrasound guidance. This chapter will review the use of ultrasound to guide pleural procedures.

Even in the hands of trained pulmonologists, supposedly experts of these procedures and the thoracic physical exam, the use of ultrasound is associated with a significant reduction in near misses (i.e., inadvertent puncture of the lung or subdiaphragmatic organs) as well as improved success rates.[1,2] Given the strength of the literature regarding ultrasound and pleural disease, the current recommendations from the British Thoracic Society recommend the use of ultrasound to guide pleural interventions, including thoracentesis and tube thoracostomy.[3]

It should be noted that most studies utilizing ultrasound for thoracentesis do not use real-time guidance for needle insertion, but rather insert the needle immediately after identification of an appropriate site. Interestingly, this "X marks the spot" technique, when performed with delay in needle insertion (having radiology use ultrasound to mark the spot, followed by needle insertion with thoracentesis being performed when the patient is returned to the floor), is not associated with

a reduction in the pneumothorax rate. A benchmark that providers and institutions should strive for is a pneumothorax rate of ~1.2%. This low rate can even be achieved in patients in the intensive care unit requiring mechanical ventilation where the "self-trained" pulmonary physician directs the house staff where to insert the needle.[4]

## PROPER POSITIONING FOR PLEURAL PROCEDURES

The initial evaluation of the patient with pleural disease should always involve the review of all available radiological imaging, as well as the patient's history and physical exam. Many inpatients receive computed tomographic imaging at some point during their stay, and if available, this type of imaging can be quite helpful in identifying size and location of pleural fluid, as well as the presence of pleural-based masses and loculations. The positioning of patients for procedures is often driven by individual patient factors. Ambulatory outpatients can be placed in a variety of positions to help facilitate procedures, whereas the ability to position a critically ill patient on a ventilator with multiple forms of life support (dialysis, ventricular assist devices, etc.) may be limited. Because of this procedural variability physicians must maintain a certain comfort level in performing ultrasound-guided pleural procedures in multiple positions and situations. In fact, the use of ultrasound allows the application of Sutton's law of the pleural space. Willie Sutton, the famous bank robber, was once asked why he robs banks. He replied, "Because that's where the money is." Ultrasound allows the operator to achieve pleural access where the "money" or, in this case, the pleural fluid is.

Before beginning any diagnostic or therapeutic procedure, it is of paramount importance to correctly identify key anatomic landmarks, including the diaphragm, parietal and visceral pleura, pleural fluid, lung, heart, aorta, spleen, liver, and kidneys.

Ultrasound examination of the pleural space should begin with identification of the diaphragm, including the presence of dynamic changes (change of shape with respiratory movement). Depending on the patient's position, the amount of pleural fluid, the presence of atelectasis or abdominal pathology, and degree of respiratory variation, the diaphragm can often be identified between the 10th and 12th rib spaces posteriorly, or the 8th and 10th rib spaces in the mid-axillary line. This, however, can change dramatically. In those patients examined in a fully recumbent position, the diaphragm can commonly be identified up into the fifth and sixth rib space. In patients with pleural fluid the diaphragm is easily identified, whereas in those patients without pleural fluid the diaphragm can only be identified through the spleen or liver.

When performing ultrasound imaging for pleural effusion on a patient's left side, it is good practice to always identify the heart and pericardium, as well as the descending thoracic aorta, prior to any procedures. The left ventricle of the heart, particularly if dilated, may be located in a very lateral position and surprisingly close to the chest wall (see Figure 4.24, page 54, and Figure 5.7, page 61).

## ERECT POSITIONING

Classic teaching for the performance of thoracentesis involves the patient sitting comfortably on the side of a bed or examination table, facing away from the examiner. The height of the bed/exam table should be adjusted so that the physician can perform the procedure in an ergonomically comfortable position (see Video 3.1, page 29). The arms of the patient should be elevated, folded across the chest, and can rest on a small bedside table placed at a comfortable height in front of him or her so as to move the scapulae laterally (Figure 9.1). This positioning should be utilized for most outpatients as well as inpatients if they are able to assume this position. Some deconditioned patients are still able to accomplish this position with the help of other support staff, using the bedside table and someone standing in front of the patient to help stabilize him or her.

The erect position allows for the most efficient and comprehensive pleural ultrasound, permitting examination of the entire posterior thorax, as well as both lateral hemithoraces (Video 9.1). If visualization of of the anterior chest is needed, simply moving to the front of the patient or even reaching around may enable the examiner to obtain the appropriate window of the anterior chest.

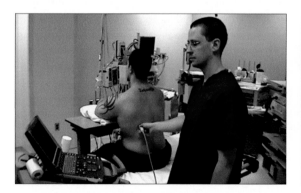

**Figure 9.1** (a) Erect positioning of patients for pleural ultrasound is ideal, and permits full access to the posterior and lateral hemithorax from a single operator position.

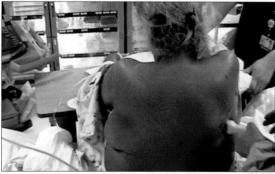

**Video 9.1** The erect position allows for the most efficient and comprehensive pleural ultrasound examination, including examination of the posterior and lateral portion of the thorax. Starting in the lower half of the hemithorax makes for quick identification of the diaphragm and potential pleural fluid. View E-book for video clip or watch it at http://goo.gl/U3xxS7.

To examine the right chest in this position, the ultrasound unit should be to the right of the examiner, so the examiner can look at his or her hand position/the position of the transducer, as well as the ultrasound screen, and manipulate the controls on the ultrasound unit with minimal effort. Likewise, the ultrasound unit should be on the examiner's left when examining the left chest.

As little as 10 ml of fluid can be visualized under ultrasound guidance with the patient in the upright position, as compared to the 150 ml of fluid that is typically needed to visualize an effusion with a standard upright phased-array (PA) and lateral chest radiograph. As free-flowing pleural effusion will accumulate in the most dependent area in the hemithorax (between the lower chest wall, the base of the lung, and the diaphragm), this is where the initial ultrasound investigations should begin.

## SUPINE POSITIONING

The supine position is most often utilized for those critically ill patients requiring bedside thoracentesis or tube thoracostomy. It is also the position traditionally taught for placement of a conventional large-bore chest tube in the mid-axillary line. Patients should be placed supine on their hospital bed with the head of the bed slightly elevated. The ipsilateral arm should be raised over the patient's head (Figure 9.2a) or brought across the chest (Figure 9.2b) and held in this position by an assistant in order to prevent contamination of the sterile field.

The semiupright supine position should also be utilized when examining the patient for pneumothorax (see Chapter 7). Elevating the head of the bed with the patient resting in a supine position will theoretically allow for free air within the thorax to rise to the most nondependent portion of the hemithorax. This will focus the area of interest to the upper portion of the anterior chest.

**Figure 9.2** To obtain pleural access in the supine patient, it is often helpful to move the ipsilateral arm above his or her head (a) or across the chest (b). The best position may be dependent on patient factors, such as inability to move a shoulder or arm. It is often helpful to have an assistant hold this arm in place.

## LATERAL AND SEMIDECUBITUS POSITIONING

Detection of pleural fluid may sometimes be difficult in the supine patient, as the location of a free-flowing effusion may vary considerably, depending upon the position of the patient, the degree of elevation of the head of the bed, as well as underlying thoracic and abdominal pathology. Though a moderate to large effusion may be visualized laterally in the supine patient, the patient may need to be rolled onto the contralateral side in order to visualize a smaller free-flowing effusion adequately (Figure 9.3). In this position, free-flowing fluid will localize nearer the spine, and care must be taken to avoid injury to the intercostal vessels, as it has been shown their course tends to be much more tortuous within 9 cm of the spinous process[5] (see Figure 4.21, page 53).

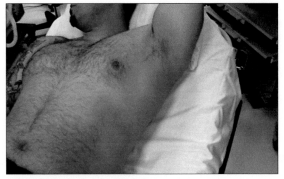

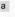
a

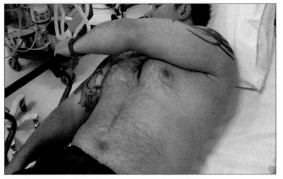
b

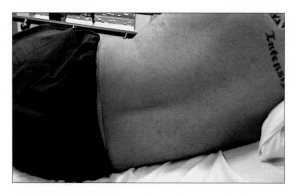

**Figure 9.3** Lateral decubitus position. It is often difficult to visualize pleural effusions under ultrasound with patients in the lateral decubitus position unless the effusions are large. Caution is advised regarding the performance of thoracentesis for small effusions in this position.

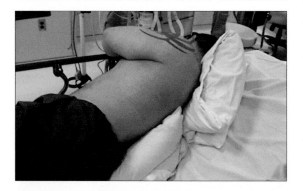

**Figure 9.4** Semilateral decubitus position. The patient's hemithorax of interest is rotated upright 30 to 45° along the axis of the spine and the ipsilateral arm elevated. This position allows for the pooling of pleural fluid toward the base of the thorax and gives the ultrasonographer access to the patient's mid-axillary or posterior axillary line.

A variation of the lateral decubitus is to utilize the semilateral decubitus position. The patient's hemithorax of interest is rotated upright 30 to 45° along the axis of the spine. The ipsilateral arm is elevated over the patient's head or across the front of the patient's torso, while the head of the bed is also elevated approximately 30°. This permits pooling of pleural fluid toward the base of the thorax and allows the ultrasonographer access to the patient's mid-axillary or posterior axillary line, where the pleural fluid may be sampled more safely. It is often useful to place a roll of towels or a folded pillow behind the patient to help maintain his or her position during the procedure (Figure 9.4).

## PLEURAL ACCESS SITE IDENTIFICATION

Most studies (and these authors) do not use real-time ultrasound guidance to visualize needle insertion, but rather ultrasound localization with pleural access immediately following identification of the appropriate access site. The selected site should be in an area that contains the largest amount of pleural fluid, while making sure mobile structures such as the lung, diaphragm, and heart do not enter the window during the respiratory cycle (see Video 3.4, page 40). Diaphragmatic excursion can be substantial even with quiet breathing and should be observed through several cycles (Video 9.2). The distance between the skin and parietal pleura, as well as the distance between the parietal pleura and lung/diaphragm, should be noted, and an image saved (Figure 9.5). The selected site should be marked using a marker or pen that will not wash off during the sterilization of the area. Alternatively, a blunt instrument may be used to make a "dent" in the skin at the intended site of pleural access (Figures 9.6a and b). The area about the mark is then prepped with chlorhexidine and draped in sterile fashion. The patient must maintain the same position after placement of the ultrasound-guided mark and should be ultrasonographically reexamined if a significant position shift or movement occurs.

## PLEURAL ACCESS FOR DIAGNOSTIC AND THERAPEUTIC ASPIRATION

Once a sterile field has been created, the skin, subcutaneous tissue, and parietal pleura are anesthetized with 1% lidocaine and a 25-gauge needle. The operator should know the tract the needle will take, based on the previously acquired ultrasound imaging (also see Video 3.4, page 40). Instead of "walking over" the rib, the authors identify the superior surface of the rib by palpation, and advance the needle in a perpendicular line just over the superior surface of the rib. After a wheal is made at the skin surface, the needle is advanced a few millimeters while maintaining suction, more lidocaine is instilled, and the process is repeated until pleural fluid or air is obtained (Videos 9.3 and 9.4). It should be noted that the parietal pleura can be quite sensitive, and should be adequately anesthetized. The visceral pleura, on the other hand, does not have pain fibers. It is imperative to follow the same angle

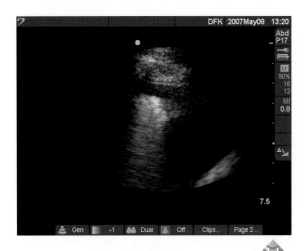

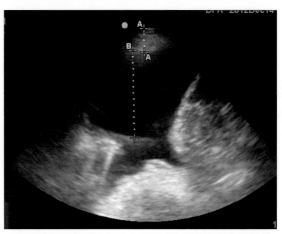

**Video 9.2** Diaphragmatic excursion can be quite substantial, even during normal respiration. This variation needs to be accounted for when planning for proper sites of pleural access. View E–book for ultrasound clip or watch it at http://goo.gl/hhDKsB.

**Figure 9.5** Ultrasound imaging noting the pathway and distance the needle will travel. The following distances are often helpful to measure and be aware of prior to beginning the procedure: skin surface to the parietal pleural surface, and surface of the parietal pleura to surface of the next closest structure, such as the lung or diaphragm.

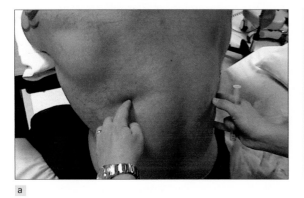

a

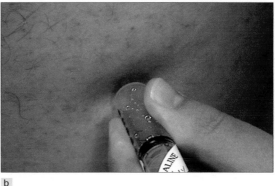

b

**Figure 9.6** Marking of the pleural access site immediately prior to needle puncture. A blunt object, including a finger (a) or a syringe (b), is used to make a dent within the skin surface. Care is taken to provide gentle pressure because this can be painful to patients, as there has usually been no anesthetic given at this point.

and orientation, with the needle corresponding to the angle and orientation of the ultrasound probe in order to minimize the risk of complications.

If fluid (or air) is not obtained, a longer needle is utilized until fluid is aspirated. In some cases (e.g., morbid obesity) a 20-gauge spinal needle can be utilized to help confirm one's ability to obtain pleural access prior to insertion of larger-gauge needles.

After local anesthesia has been achieved, in the case of a diagnostic thoracentesis, once enough fluid is

collected for appropriate sampling, the needle can be withdrawn and the procedure terminated. The same holds true when performing simple aspiration for pneumothorax.

When performing a therapeutic thoracentesis, the technique will vary depending on which equipment is used/available to perform the procedure. The authors will detail use of a thoracentesis kit here. After local anesthesia has been achieved, a 4 mm skin incision is made parallel to and overlying the superior surface

CHAPTER 9

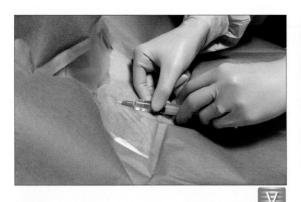

**Video 9.3** Local anesthesia is provided with a 25-gauge finder needle. An initial wheal at the access site should be performed. View E-book for video clip or watch it at http://goo.gl/AXa629.

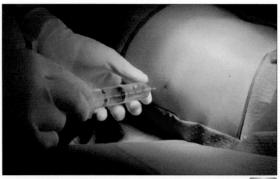

**Video 9.4** The same 25-gauge finder needle is utilized for further chest wall anesthesia. The needle is advanced as further anesthesia is provided. This cycle continues to repeat itself until the parietal pleura is reached. The ability to freely aspirate pleural fluid confirms entrance into the pleural space. View E-book for video clip or watch it at http://goo.gl/ETcAYM.

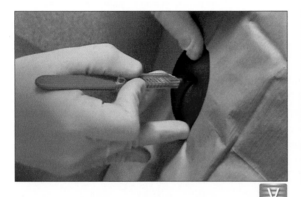

**Video 9.5** A small stab incision (approximately 4 mm) is made to allow for easy access and advancement of the larger thoracentesis needle and catheter. View E-book for video clip or watch it at http://goo.gl/rl1wMY.

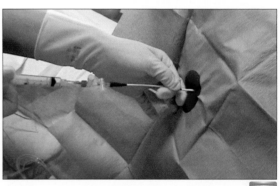

**Video 9.6** Utilizing the thoracentesis catheter–needle assembly and the previous needle path, the entire unit is advanced until pleural fluid is obtained. Once the presence of free-flowing pleural fluid is confirmed, the catheter is then advanced over the needle into the pleural space. View E-book for video clip or watch it at http://goo.gl/p06Ay1.

of the rib (Video 9.5). A perpendicular incision is not made, due to the risk of transecting one of the intercostal vessels. Clearly, the orientation of the incision will change depending on the patient's position, and will not be parallel to the floor in a supine patient. At this point an 8 French thoracentesis catheter over the needle is introduced through the skin incision and same needle tract, while maintaining negative pressure on the syringe. Once fluid is obtained in the syringe, the catheter is advanced over the needle and the needle removed (Video 9.6). The authors prefer the use of a syringe-pump connected system as opposed to using a vacuum bottle, as the latter has been associated with an increased risk of pneumothorax,[6] and the syringe-pump system easily allows for the measurement of pleural pressures.[7]

If a sterile sheath is available, ultrasound can be performed intermittently throughout the pleural drainage to confirm lung expansion. Otherwise, repeat ultrasound can be performed at the termination of the procedure to both confirm lung expansion and rule out pneumothorax.

## PLEURAL ACCESS FOR INTERCOSTAL TUBE DRAINAGE

Patient positioning for intercostal tube drainage can involve any of the aforementioned positions, though the authors tend to insert the tubes posterior–laterally for effusions, and either anterior–laterally (fifth intercostal space in the mid-axillary line) or anteriorly (second to third intercostal space in the mid-clavicular line) for pneumothorax. If inserting the tube anteriorly, care should be taken to avoid the internal mammary artery, as well as the subclavian vessels.

The use of small-bore intercostal tubes (≤14 French) has increased in popularity due to equivalent drainage, as well as decreased pain both during insertion and while in place, when compared with larger tubes for most pleural effusions (including empyema) or pneumothorax.[8] Although still debated, some authors would recommend larger-bore chest tubes for the management of hemothorax and large continuous air leaks.

The insertion of most small-bore intercostal drains utilizes the modified Seldinger technique. After proper positioning, sterilization, and appropriate draping, as mentioned above, pleural access should initially be obtained with a small finder needle. Once the ability to aspirate pleural fluid (or air) is confirmed and the tract anesthetized, a 4 mm skin incision should be made—again parallel to the rib. This incision will make for easier over-the-wire tract dilation.

An introducer needle is then inserted into the pleural space, again confirming the free aspiration of pleural fluid or air. The syringe is removed, and a guide wire introduced through the needle (Video 9.7). The guide wire should advance easily, without force, as the inability to easily advance the guide wire may suggest misplacement of the needle, potentially leading to the creation of a subcutaneous false tract or, worse, puncture of other surrounding organs. After the guide wire has been advanced, the needle is removed and a dilator is introduced. Easy manipulation of the wire at this stage will confirm that it hasn't kinked over the rib during dilation (Video 9.8). Once the tract has been dilated, the dilator is removed and the intercostal tube can be advanced over the guide wire. The tube is advanced into position and the stiffener and guide wire removed together (Video 9.9). This tube is sutured into place and connected to a chest tube drainage system, with the application of thoracic suction as appropriate to the indication for tube placement.

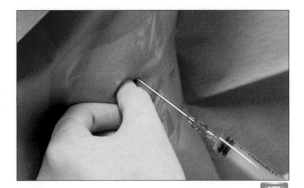

**Video 9.7** Access to the pleural space is again confirmed with the 18-gauge introducer needle. After confirmation of free-flowing pleural fluid, the syringe is removed and the guide wire is quickly introduced. The guide wire should pass easily. Any difficulty in passage of the wire should prompt consideration for repositioning of the needle or reevaluation of the access site. View E-book for video clip or watch it at http://goo.gl/ccjCm8.

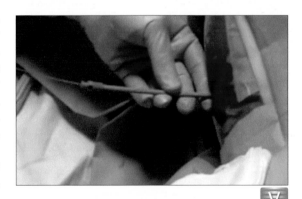

**Video 9.8** The tract dilator is next introduced over the guide wire. The dilator should easily pass over the guide wire, as difficulty in passing may indicate bending of the guide wire and the potential creation of a false tract. The proper positioning can also be confirmed by moving the guide wire back and forth, as this will confirm you remain in the original tract you created. View E-book for video clip or watch it at http://goo.gl/vmLdpw.

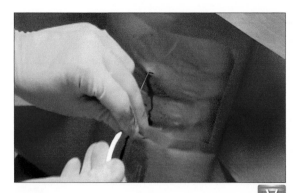

**Video 9.9** The thoracostomy tube and stiffener are introduced over the guide wire, and using the Seldinger technique the tube is passed until it enters the pleural space. At that point the guide wire and stiffener are secured with one hand and the tube advanced over them into the pleural space. View E-book for video clip or watch it at http://goo.gl/X8CuwV.

Conventional, larger-bore straight chest tubes can also be placed under guidance of ultrasound either with the modified Seldinger technique or with blunt (surgical) dissection. Though access of the pleural space is confirmed by the operator's finger when using surgical dissection, ultrasound should be used to help localize the appropriate intercostal space for pleural access. It will also provide information on the presence of lung tethered to the pleural surface, so highlighting areas to avoid for tube insertion (see Figure 6.9, page 77).

## REAL-TIME ULTRASOUND-GUIDED PLEURAL PROCEDURES

Pleural access can also be obtained under real-time ultrasound visualization. There is currently no data available to suggest that this technique offers improved safety or efficacy when compared to performing pleural ultrasound immediately prior to the procedure. The proposed advantages to using this technique include the real-time visualization of the needle as it enters the target. This has the potential to improve yield and reduce complications by avoiding surrounding structures when accessing a small or complex effusion. The disadvantages include awkwardness of holding both needle and probe while attempting to locate target, the technique requires more time, skill (specifically hand–eye coordination), and practice, and requires specific equipment (sterile ultrasound gel and probe sheath).

If real-time ultrasound guidance is used, the ultrasound probe can be orientated in the transverse (Figure 9.7) or longitudinal (Figure 9.8) axis and the procedure performed using the in-plane or out-of-plane method, respectively. The out-of-plane technique (Video 9.10) is often favored as the easier of the two, but care must be taken not to misinterpret the shaft of the needle as the needle tip. The needle tip is identified when the needle disappears by increasing tilt angle of the probe (see Video 9.10).

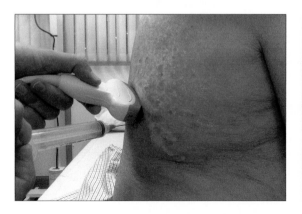

**Figure 9.7** Real-time ultrasound-guided aspiration using the in-plane technique. The probe is held in the transverse axis with the needle inserted at the edge of the probe. The needle is advanced along the intercostal space so the entire needle path is kept in view until the pleural space is reached.

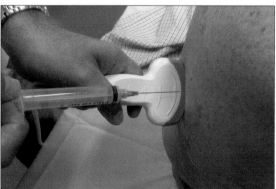

**Figure 9.8** Real-time ultrasound-guided aspiration using the out-of-plane technique. The probe is held in the longitudinal axis and the needle inserted at the mid-point of the probe and advanced to enter the pleural space (see Video 9.10, page 119).

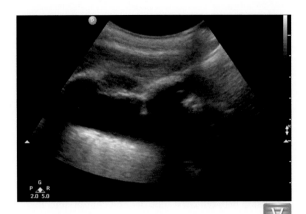

**Video 9.10** Real-time ultrasound-guided pleural aspiration using the out-of-plane technique, with the probe in longitudinal orientation. (Courtesy of Dr. James Rippey.) View E-book for video clip or watch it at http://goo.gl/xsTBgM.

The in-plane technique during real-time performance allows imaging of the entire needle path, but a shallower needle angle of entry is required, meaning a greater distance of chest wall is traversed before the pleural space is reached. This increased distance to target can cause difficulties, especially in the obese patient. The ultrasound plane for a typical 12 mHz linear probe is approximately 1 mm thick, so good hand–eye coordination is required to keep the entire needle in that correct plane using this technique.

Regardless of which method is used, experience is required to perform the procedure adequately. In the right hands, real-time ultrasound needlework has the potential to be safer. A tip for the beginner is to start practicing with larger effusions to help develop competence and dexterity prior to tackling smaller targets. Equipment to aid real-time guided procedures is also available; needle guides attach onto the ultrasound probe to keep the needle in the correct plane, and echogenic needles allow the needle (or tip) to be more easily identified on ultrasound.

## OTHER USES FOR ULTRASOUND-GUIDED PLEURAL ACCESS

Pleural ultrasound should also be utilized to assist with the insertion of all indwelling or tunneled pleural catheters (TPCs) and guide insertion sites for medical thoracoscopy. For both of these procedures, the patient is placed in the lateral decubitus position, with the affected side uppermost. For the placement of TPCs, the authors favor a more inferior and lateral location for pleural access, understanding that after drainage of the effusion, the diaphragm may achieve a more superior position in the thorax. Trocar insertion sites for medical thoracoscopy depend on the indication for the procedure. For the diagnosis of malignant pleural disease, a more inferior site is selected, as tumor nodules tend to occupy the inferior posterior pleura, whereas the fifth intercostal space is typically the preferred site for the management of pneumothorax.

## CONCLUSION

The use of ultrasonography has revolutionized access to the pleural space, and is associated with a significant reduction in complications from commonly performed pleural procedures. It is important that operators utilize a standard approach to both ultrasound examinations of the pleural space and the procedures they will perform, and receive dedicated draining in both of these components of pleural procedures.

### TIPS FOR CLINICAL PRACTICE

- The use of pleural ultrasound offers many advantages over traditional thoracentesis, including improved safety, efficacy, and decreased incidence of dry taps.

- The erect position remains the preferred position for the performance of pleural fluid aspiration; however, clinical situations may dictate otherwise, and clinicians should remain facile at performing procedures in other positions.

- When performing pleural aspiration (for fluid or air), follow Sutton's law of the pleural space, i.e., go where the money is. Be mindful, however, of the potential increased risk of intercostal artery laceration with more medial approaches.

- Pleural ultrasound can be used to help facilitate placement of indwelling pleural catheters as well as aiding in the identification of appropriate trocar insertion sites for medical thoracoscopy.

CHAPTER 9

CHAPTER 9

## REFERENCES

1. Diacon AH, Brutsche MH, Soler M. Accuracy of pleural puncture sites: a prospective comparison of clinical examination with ultrasound. *Chest* 2003; 123(2):436–441.

2. Gordon CE, Feller-Kopman D, Balk EM, Smetana GW. Pneumothorax following thoracentesis: a systematic review and meta-analysis. *Archives of Internal Medicine* 2010; 170(4):332–339.

3. Havelock T, Teoh R, Laws D, Gleeson F. Pleural procedures and thoracic ultrasound: British Thoracic Society pleural disease guideline 2010. *Thorax* 2010; 65:i61–i76.

4. Mayo PH, Goltz HR, Tafreshi M, Doelken P. Safety of ultrasound-guided thoracentesis in patients receiving mechanical ventilation. *Chest* 2004; 125(3):1059–1062.

5. Yoneyama H, Arahata M, Temaru R, Ishizaka S, Minami S. Evaluation of the risk of intercostal artery laceration during thoracentesis in elderly patients by using 3D-CT angiography. *Internal Medicine* 2010; 49(4):289–292.

6. Petersen WG, Zimmerman R. Limited utility of chest radiograph after thoracentesis. *Chest* 2000; 117(4):1038–1042.

7. Feller-Kopman D, Parker MJ, Schwartzstein RM. Assessment of pleural pressure in the evaluation of pleural effusions. *Chest* 2009; 135(1):201–209.

8. Rahman NM, Maskell NA, Davies CWH et al. The relationship between chest tube size and clinical outcome in pleural infection. *Chest* 2010; 137(3):536–543.

### MCQ 1

**Q** The ideal patient position for thoracentesis is:

**a.** Lateral decubitus.

**b.** Erect, sitting on the side of the bed.

**c.** Supine.

**d.** Lithotomy position.

### MCQ 2

**Q** Thoracic ultrasound can be useful in all of the following situations, except:

**a.** Aspiration of pleural fluid.

**b.** Needle aspiration of pleural-based mass.

**c.** Needle aspiration of a solitary pulmonary nodule.

**d.** Guidance for insertion sites for medical thoracoscopy.

### MCQ 3

**Q** The presence of an echo-free space on pleural ultrasound always confirms the presence of pleural fluid.

**a.** True.

**b.** False.

### MCQ 4

**Q** The use of thoracic ultrasound for thoracentesis does not help improve the safety or efficacy of the procedure in expert hands.

**a.** True.

**b.** False.

### ANSWERS

 **1.** b

 **2.** c

The pathology must be visualized to be suitable for biopsy. A solitary pulmonary nodule will not be seen on thoracic ultrasound when surrounded by normal aerated lung

 **3.** b

Other structures and pathology can be seen as an echo-free space, including the heart (cardiac chambers containing anechoic blood) and pleural thickening. See Chapter 9 for further detail.

 **4.** b

See Chapters 1 and 9.

# Ultrasound Skills and Application Beyond the Pleura

Coenraad F.N. Koegelenberg and Andreas H. Diacon

## INTRODUCTION

Transthoracic ultrasonography is a well-established modality in the evaluation of respiratory disorders, but has significant potential beyond diagnosis of pleural and lung disorders. Although healthy lung parenchyma cannot be visualized by ultrasound, many indications for the use of this modality beyond the pleura have been validated in the last few decades. These include the assessment and guidance of biopsy of extrathoracic lymph nodes, chest wall (including skeletal) pathology, and consolidating pulmonary diseases that abut the chest wall and anterior mediastinal masses. Transthoracic ultrasound has many advantages that make it an ideal investigation in these settings, including its immediate application, mobility, the fact that it utilizes no radiation, and its short examination time. Moreover, ultrasound-assisted biopsy can be performed by a single clinician with no sedation and minimal monitoring, even potentially outside of theatre.[1–3]

Basic two-dimensional ultrasound equipment provides adequate images for the indications described in this chapter, and the use of M mode or color flow Doppler is very rarely indicated for the applications discussed in this chapter. Specific reusable probes for real-time ultrasound guidance of needle biopsies are commercially available, but most clinicians use the freehand technique to perform ultrasound-assisted biopsy.

## EXTRATHORACIC LYMPH NODES

*Cervical, supraclavicular*, and *axillary lymph nodes* are accessible with ultrasound, and ultrasound may aid in distinguishing reactive from malignant lymph nodes. Inflammatory lymph nodes have an echogenic fatty hilum and oval or triangular shapes, compared to malignant nodes, which are often bulky and show loss of the fatty hilum, leading to a hypoechoic appearance (Figure 10.1a). Irregular borders are suggestive of extracapsular spread.

Ultrasound-guided fine-needle aspiration (FNA) of supraclavicular lymph nodes is standard practice in many institutions, and has the advantage of providing a cytological diagnosis and pathological staging (pN3) in one minimally invasive procedure. A recent report highlighted the usefulness of ultrasound-guided FNA of supraclavicular lymph nodes: The procedure provided pathological diagnoses in 18.7% (95% CI = 15.9–20.5%) of all cases of lung cancer diagnosed over a 2-year period (n = 996).[4] Ultrasound has the added advantage that it can be used to visualize cervical or supraclavicular lymph nodes in patients who present with superior vena cava obstruction, particularly when swelling and vascular congestion complicate routine physical palpation (Figure 10.1b—clip).

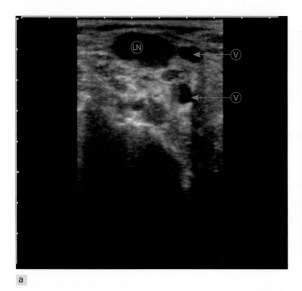

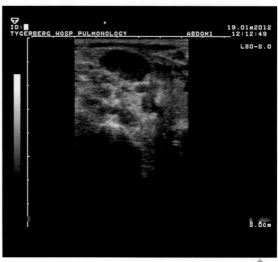

a

b

**Figure 10.1** (a) High-frequency ultrasound view showing a large cervical lymph node (LN) with surrounding tissue edema and distended vessels (V) in a patient who presented with superior vena cava syndrome secondary to small cell lung cancer. Ultrasound was used to guide aspiration of this lymph node and to confirm the diagnosis in this particular case. (b) Video of (a). The probe is moved in cephalad and caudad. Note the large lymph node is only observed in certain planes (and therefore changes shape and disappears), whereas the surrounding distended veins and (pulsating) arteries remain visible throughout. View E-book for ultrasound clip or watch it at http://goo.gl/ILzkkD.

## CHEST WALL AND SKELETAL PATHOLOGY

High-frequency ultrasound can detect *soft-tissue masses* (Figure 10.2) with ease, and even *bony metastases* to the ribs (Figure 10.3), which appear as hypoechoic masses replacing the normal echogenicity of a rib and leading to the disruption of the cortical line. Furthermore, ultrasound has even been shown to be more sensitive than radiography in the detection of rib fracture, which appears as a breach or displacement of the rib cortex with or without a localized swelling or hematoma.

Chest wall masses and thoracic bony metastases are well suited for transthoracic ultrasound-assisted biopsy, as no aerated lung needs to be transversed during biopsy (Figure 10.4—clip). Ultrasound-assisted transthoracic fine-needle aspiration (TTFNA) is performed under local anesthesia, ideally with a 22-G injection-type or short (pediatric) spinal needle with a removable inner stylet (to reduce contamination with chest wall tissue and blood), connected to a 10-ml syringe. Cutting needle biopsy (CNB) follows the same principles as TTFNA, but the devices are more invasive and carry a higher risk of vascular or visceral trauma.

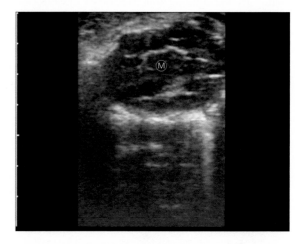

**Figure 10.2** High-frequency ultrasound of a soft-tissue chest wall mass (M) (plasmacytoma). Note the internal echoes, hyperechoic distal margin, and reverberation artifacts, all indicative of a mass with a high fluid content.

Great care must be taken not to inadvertently pass these devices through the ribs (and potentially cause visceral trauma), as osteolytic rib metastases may offer less resistance than expected (similar to soft tissue).

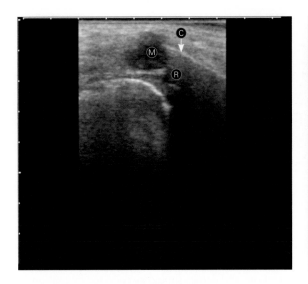

**Figure 10.3** High-frequency ultrasound of a metastatic deposit (M) in the dorsal aspect of a rib (R). Note the hypoechoic appearance of the metastasis and the disruption of the normal cortical line (C).

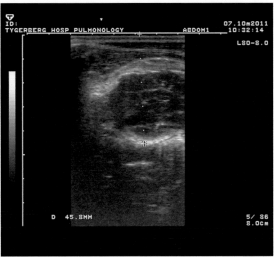

**Figure 10.4** High-frequency ultrasound view of a patient with a plasmacytoma on whom an ultrasound-assisted fine-needle aspiration and Tru-Cut biopsy were performed. The depth of interest is measured (and intended direction of FNA memorized), whereafter the FNA is performed freehand. View E-book for ultrasound clip or watch it at http://goo.gl/iXbzo3.

## PULMONARY PATHOLOGY

### Lung tumors

Provided aerated lung tissue is replaced by consolidated or solid lung tissue and pleural contact is present, practically any pathological processes become detectable with ultrasound. Lung tumors often appear hypoechoic with posterior acoustic enhancement and irregular borders.

Note that the acoustic window is invariably too narrow to demonstrate the whole circumference of the lesion, but it allows an accurate determination of the depth (Figure 10.5). High-resolution ultrasound scanning is superior to routine chest computed tomography (CT) in evaluating tumor invasion of the pleura and chest

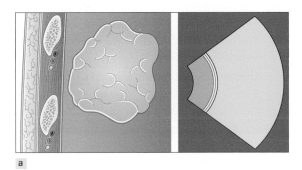

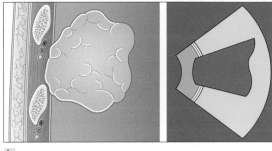

a                                                          b

**Figure 10.5** A peripheral lung lesion is shown schematically on the left, without (a) and with (b) pleural contact. The corresponding sonar images recorded with a sector scanner are shown on the right. Only the lesion with pleural contact is visible on ultrasound. Note that the acoustic window is too narrow to demonstrate the whole circumference of the lesion, but it allows determination of its full depth. (Adapted with permission from: Diacon AH, Theron J, Bolliger CT. Transthoracic ultrasound for the pulmonologist. *Curr Opin Pulm.)*

wall, which has a direct impact on tumor staging (T2 or T3 staging, respectively). The visceral pleural line is interrupted once the visceral pleura is infiltrated (Figure 10.6), whereas loss of movement with respiration on low- or high-frequency scanning is indicative of extension beyond the parietal pleura (Figure 10.7—clip). Associated pulmonary collapse may cause fluid bronchograms.[2]

Most clinicians utilize the "freehand" technique for ultrasound-assisted biopsy of pulmonary tumors, and both ultrasound-assisted TTFNA and CNB may be employed (Figure 10.8). Following appropriate patient positioning, the intended site of needle insertion is identified with ultrasound and marked, while the direction, depth of interest, and safety range for the procedure are determined (Figures 10.9 and 10.10—clips).[1,2] It is essential that the patient must not alter position in order to prevent a positional shift of the area of interest relative to the skin mark. TTFNA can be performed with 22-G spinal needles (40 mm or 90 mm) in length (as needed) connected to a 10-ml syringe under sterile conditions with local anesthesia (1% lignocaine). While applying approximately 5 ml of negative pressure, aspirates from at least four slightly different directions and depths should be collected by cautiously moving the needle in and out within the predetermined (measured) safety range. The material should immediately be expressed onto slides and fixed or stained within seconds. Where available, rapid on-site evaluation (ROSE) of the cytology specimens should be employed to assess the need for CNB in the same setting. CNB caries a higher risk of visceral injury and pneumothorax, and should only be used if a sufficient

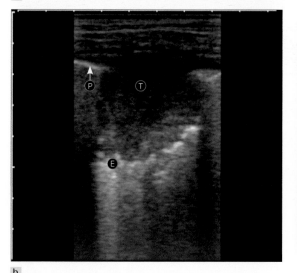

a

b

**Figure 10.6** A peripheral lung tumor. Note the CT appearance (a) and corresponding high-frequency ultrasound image (b). The acoustic window is too narrow to demonstrate the whole circumference of the lesion, but it allows determination of its full depth. The lung tumor (T) is infiltrating the chest wall. Note the peripheral acoustic enhancement (E) and the disruption of the visceral and parietal pleural (P).

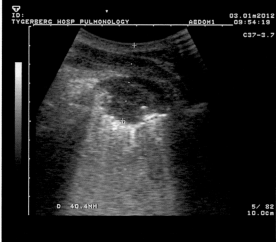

**Figure 10.7** Low-frequency ultrasound view of a patient with peripheral lung tumor with chest wall invasion. Note the loss of the pleural lines and specifically the loss of movement with respiration. Also note how the depth of the ultrasound is adjusted in order to better visualize the tumor and calculate the safety range. View E-book for ultrasound clip or watch it at http://goo.gl/DFj1xC.

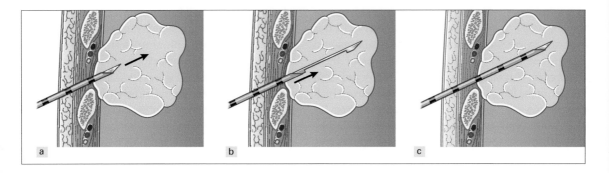

**Figure 10.8** Tru-Cut biopsy of a peripheral lung tumor with chest wall invasion. (a) The device is positioned within the lesion, keeping a safe distance from the intercostal neurovascular structures below the ribs. (b) The inner stylet is deployed with the cutting bit pointing away from the neurovascular bundle. (c) The biopsy specimen is harvested by sliding the cutting bit over the inner stylet (not by withdrawing the inner stylet back into the cutting bit). The absence of air between the lung lesion and the chest wall provides both an acoustic window and a pathway for the sampling device through nonaerated tissue, which reduces the risk of pneumothorax. (Adapted with permission from: Diacon AH, Theron J, Bolliger CT. Transthoracic ultrasound for the pulmonologist. *Curr Opin Pulm.*)

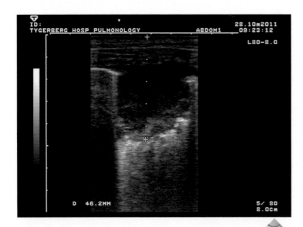

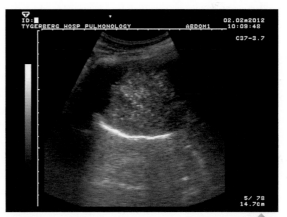

**Figure 10.9** High-frequency ultrasound view of a patient with peripheral lung tumor with chest wall invasion. Note how the path and depth of the intended fine-needle aspiration are measured, whereafter the procedure is performed freehand. View E-book for ultrasound clip or watch it at http://goo.gl/cm98sL.

**Figure 10.10** A low-frequency ultrasound view of a patient with large peripheral lung tumor with chest wall invasion. One again, note how the path and depth of the intended fine-needle aspiration are measured, whereafter the procedure is performed freehand. In this particular case, small cell lung cancer was diagnosed by means of TTFNA. View E-book for ultrasound clip or watch it at http://goo.gl/ox6RYt.

safety range can be assured (i.e., there is no major blood vessel or organ close to the intended CNB path). Ultrasound should also routinely be used to assess the pleural space for the presence of a pneumothorax following TTFNA and CNB (see Chapter 7).

The authors have found that ultrasound-assisted CNB has a sensitivity of approximately 85% for lung tumors abutting the chest wall and 100% for meso-thelioma.[5] CNB is safe, with a pneumothorax rate

of 4%. In a more recent study, we found ultrasound-assisted TTFNA with ROSE by a cytopathologist to have a yield of 82% in the setting of tumors abutting the chest wall. CNB was shown to be diagnostic in 76%, and the combined yield of CNB and TTFNA was 89%.[6] Both ultrasound-guided CNB and FNA had a low complication rate, with pneumothoraces observed in 4% and 1.3%, respectively.[6] Subanalyses showed that ultrasound-guided TTFNA was superior to CNB in confirming a diagnosis of epithelial carcinomas of the lung (95% vs. 81%, $p = 0.006$), whereas CNB was superior in cases of noncarcinomatous tumors and benign lesions. The practical implications of these findings are that ultrasound-assisted TTFNA and CNB are safe in the hands of clinicians, that both have a high diagnostic yield, and that CNB may be reserved for cases where cytology is noncontributory and a diagnosis other than epithelial carcinoma of the lung cancer is suspected.

## Pulmonary consolidation

Ultrasound may also be used in the detection and sampling of pulmonary consolidation. Pneumonic consolidation (Figure 10.11) often appears less extensive on ultrasound than on chest radiographs. Early on the parenchyma appears diffusely echogenic, similar to the ultrasonographic texture of the liver.[1] Both air and fluid bronchograms may be observed within the consolidated lung (Figure 10.12—clip). Air bronchograms appear as echogenic branches and echogenic foci that fluctuate with respiration.[1] Fluid bronchograms represent fluid-filled airways that are seen as anechoic

tubular structures, and may be associated with bronchial obstruction or extensive pneumonic consolidation. Furthermore, ultrasound is ideally suited to differentiate dense consolidation from pleural effusions in critically ill patients (Figures 10.13 and 10.14), and to guide thoracocentesis in the same setting (see Chapter 9). Consolidation may also be observed with bronchial obstruction, pulmonary infarction, hemorrhage, bronchoalveolar carcinoma, and numerous other noninfectious disease processes. Ultrasound-assisted TTFNA of consolidated lung secondary to pneumonia is infrequently performed in everyday practice, but is safe and has a high diagnostic yield with respect to the confirmation of the offending pathogen. The microbiological yield of ultrasound-assisted biopsy of pulmonary consolidation of unknown etiology is higher than 90%, and ultrasound-assisted TTFNA can be particularly useful in immunocompromised and critically ill patients. Ultrasound should routinely be used to assess for the presence of a pneumothorax following TTFNA, particularly in ventilated patients. Prospective studies of consolidation biopsy are required to assess the general clinical applicability.

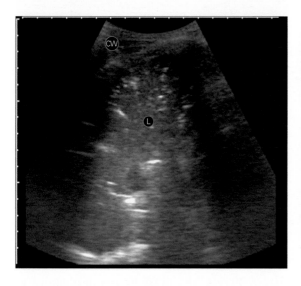

**Figure 10.11** A low-frequency ultrasound image of a densely consolidated lung (L) abutting the chest wall (CW). Note the multiple echogenic air bronchograms (best seen on real-time video imaging—Figure 10.12).

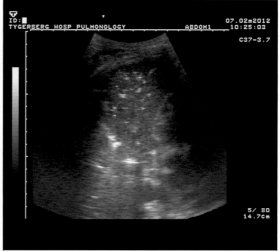

**Figure 10.12** Low-frequency ultrasound view of a patient with pneumonia. Note the multiple dynamic echogenic foci (air bronchograms) and hypoechoic branching fluid bronchograms. View E-book for ultrasound clip or watch it at http://goo.gl/N5s9OT.

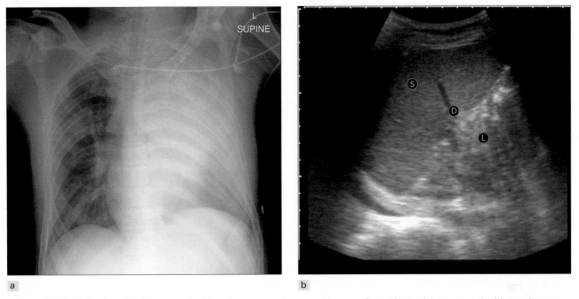

**Figure 10.13** (a) Supine chest x-ray, and (b) low-frequency ultrasound image of a patient who presented with respiratory failure and a densely consolidated left lung. Note the absence of pleural fluid and the dense consolidation (L) on ultrasound. The diaphragm (D) and spleen (S) can be seen.

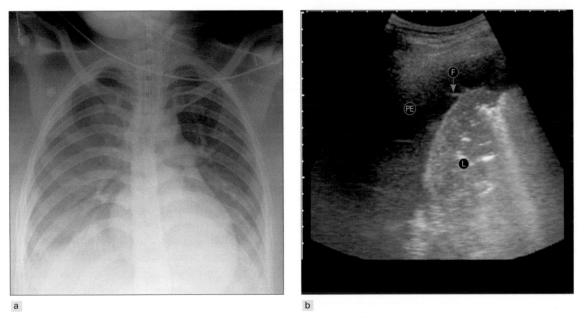

**Figure 10.14** (a) Supine chest x-ray, and (b) low-frequency ultrasound image of a second patient who presented with respiratory failure. Note the presence of a pleural effusion (PE) with fibrin strands (F) and the partially atelectatic, densely consolidated lung (L) on ultrasound.

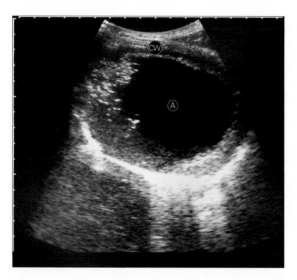

**Figure 10.15** Low-frequency ultrasound image of a lung abscess (A) abutting the chest wall (CW). Note the irregular margin and the hyperechoic distal wall.

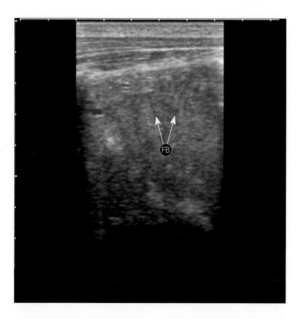

**Figure 10.16** This high-frequency ultrasound shows fluid bronchograms (FB) as anechoic tubular structures inside the drowned lung.

## Lung abscesses

A lung abscess that abuts the chest wall pleura appears as a hypoechoic lesion with a well-defined or irregular wall (Figure 10.15). The center of the abscess is most often anechoic, but septations and internal echoes may be seen. Abscesses with air fluid levels are more inhomogeneous and change in appearance as the patient changes from a sitting to a supine position. The vast majority of lung abscesses are visible on ultrasound, and the TTFNA is more than 90% likely to be diagnostic for a specific pathogen, although pleural contamination remains a potential complication. Again, prospective studies on ultrasound-assisted pulmonary abscess aspiration are required to assess its real clinical usefulness and complication rate.

## Drowned lung

Lung tumors are not usually discernible on ultrasound, but may cause varying degrees of pulmonary collapse (resorptive atelectasis) and post-obstructive pneumonitis. "Drowned lung" is a radiological term often used to describe these areas that are considered to represent accumulated secretions, and typified on CT by enhanced pulmonary vasculature contrasted against surrounding pulmonary consolidation. It is detectable on ultrasound, and typified by fluid bronchograms, provided the consolidation extends to the chest wall (Figure 10.16). In a recent study, the authors found that ultrasound-assisted TTFNA from drowned lung was diagnostic in 74.2% of cases, and represented a viable alternative to bronchoscopy in some patients.[7] Moreover, we observed no pneumothoraces, as no aerated lung was transversed.

## The breathless patient

Transthoracic ultrasound may be utilized to evaluate the breathless patient, and specifically to differentiate pulmonary edema and other alveolar–interstitial syndromes from a chronic obstructive airway disease.[8] Normal lung parenchyma cannot be visualized on transthoracic ultrasound.[1–3,10] The large change in acoustic impedance at the pleura–lung interface, however, results in horizontal artifacts that are seen as a series of echogenic parallel lines equidistant from one another below the pleura, known as reverberation artifacts or A lines. Vertical comet-tail artifacts, caused by fluid-filled subpleural interlobular septae, can be seen originating at the pleura–lung interface in

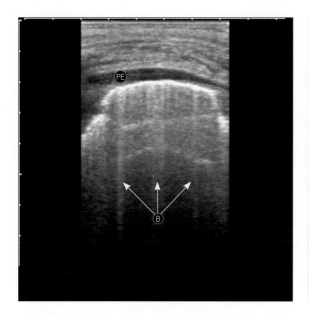

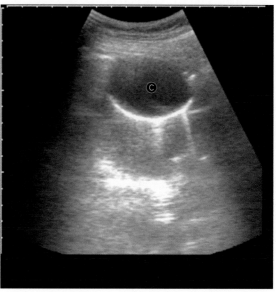

**Figure 10.17** This high-frequency ultrasound shows multiple B lines (B), as well as a small pleural effusion (PE), in a patient with pulmonary edema secondary to mitral stenosis.

**Figure 10.18** A low-frequency ultrasound showing a cyst (C). Note the distal hyperechoic wall and reverberation artifact, both secondary to the high fluid content.

normal individuals, and are best seen at the lung bases. Long, well-defined comet tails that obliterate A lines are referred to as B lines (Figure 10.17). The presence of multiple B lines (referred to as "lung rockets") in the setting of patients with acute dyspnea has been reported to be a reliable sign favoring pulmonary edema. Lichtenstein and co-workers found that B lines were absent in 92% of patients with chronic obstructive airway disease, but present in 93% of patients with alveolar–interstitial syndromes.[9]

## Pulmonary embolism

More sophisticated applications of transthoracic ultrasound include the assessment of patients with possible pulmonary embolism. Pulmonary infarction may be visualized as a peripheral wedge-shaped hypoechoic region, frequently accompanied by an effusion. A central hyperechoic bronchiole and a congested pulmonary vessel may be observed. The extent of pulmonary infarction is underappreciated on ultrasound. In experienced hands, thoracic ultrasound has a reported sensitivity of 77–89% and specificity of 66–83% for pulmonary embolism. In reality, however, CT angiography remains the investigation of choice, albeit ultrasound in experienced hands may contribute more widely to illuminate the clinical picture of thromboembolic disease by demonstrating right ventricular overload and liver congestion in case of pulmonary embolism or noncompressible deep veins, suggesting thrombosis all in one.

## Other indications

Other indications for the use of transthoracic ultrasound include the assessment and guided aspiration of pulmonary and pleural-based *cysts* (e.g., hydatid disease). These cysts can be visualized as large, round anechoic lesions (Figure 10.18). *Rounded atelectasis* may be visualized as a pleural-based mass with associated pleural thickening and extrapleural fat. The invaginated pleura may result in an echogenic line running from the pleura into the mass. *Pulmonary arteriovenous malformations* appear as distinct hypoechoic lesions with posterior acoustic enhancement. Lesions display high vascularity on Doppler, with low-impedance flow.

## MEDIASTINAL PATHOLOGY

The differential diagnosis of mediastinal masses is broad, and CT scanning followed by biopsy is performed in practically all cases. Mediastinoscopy, mediastinotomy, or related surgical procedures are currently the most popular ways of harvesting tissue. These procedures have diagnostic yields in excess of 90%, but are associated with a complication rate of up to 5% and have to be performed in theatre under general anesthesia.

Ultrasound-assisted biopsy of mediastinal masses (Figure 10.19) provides a significantly less invasive, safer, and cheaper alternative to mediastinoscopy or mediastinotomy.[10] The technique is comparable to that of ultrasound-assisted biopsy of lung masses, but even extra attention needs to be given to identifying a safe biopsy tract, given the vicinity of the heart and great vessels (Figure 10.20—clip). Furthermore, mediastinal structures may be significantly displaced in the diseased state.

In a landmark study from the late 1980s, Saito and co-workers[11] diagnosed 31 of 45 mediastinal masses by means of ultrasound-guided needle biopsies. In total, 13 of 15 patients with malignancies had diagnostic biopsies. Yang et al.[12] subsequently found Tru-Cut needles to have a diagnostic yield of 88.9% for mediastinal tumors. The same author also pioneered the supraclavicular approach for ultrasound-guided biopsies of superior mediastinal tumors. Despite these encouraging findings, ultrasound-assisted mediastinal biopsy has not gained popularity among clinicians, possibly because investigators generally utilized only the more invasive CNB option and were almost exclusively specialist interventional radiologists. Studies that included more than 40 patients reported a 1–6% complication rate from CNB, with pneumothoraces, hemothoraces, and hemoptysis the most common serious complications.

CHAPTER 10

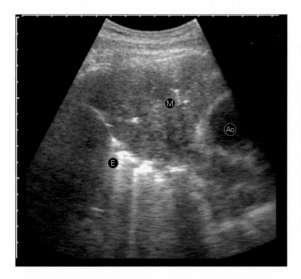

**Figure 10.19** This low-frequency image of an anterior mediastinal mass (M) was obtained from a right parasternal approach. Note the posterior enhancement (E) and the descending aorta (Ao).

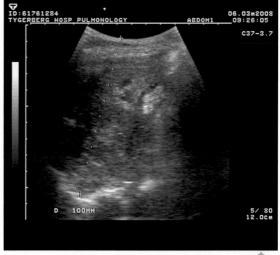

**Figure 10.20** Low-frequency ultrasound view of a paracardiac mediastinal mass. Note how the angle of the intended biopsy path is estimated and how a safety range is maintained. View E- book for ultrasound clip or watch it at http://goo.gl/u36XBg.

In a recent study the authors performed ultrasound-assisted TTFNA with ROSE on 45 consecutive patients, immediately followed by CNB only, where a provisional diagnosis of epithelial carcinoma or tuberculosis could not be established and a clear safety range of at least 1cm could be ensured.[10] An accurate cytological diagnosis was made in 33 (73.3%), and was more likely to be diagnostic in epithelial carcinoma and tuberculosis than all other pathology ($p < 0.001$). CNB was only needed in a minority of cases and yielded a diagnosis in 88.2%. Overall, 93.3% of patients were diagnosed in a single session.

In an earlier study, we performed ultrasound-assisted biopsy on 25 consecutive patients with SVC syndrome with an associated mass lesion that abutted the chest wall. TTFNA had a diagnostic yield of 96%, and ultrasound-assisted CNB a diagnostic yield of 87.5%. The incidence of minor hemorrhage was 4% following TTFNA and 18.8% following CNB. Neither procedure resulted in major hemorrhage or pneumothoraces.

## TIPS FOR CLINICAL PRACTICE

1. Appreciate that peripheral lymph nodes, chest wall pathology, anterior mediastinal masses, and consolidating pulmonary pathology that abut the chest wall are discernible on transthoracic ultrasound.

2. Take time to position the patient adequately (after surveying all available imaging modalities). This may include rotating the scapulae out of the way.

3. Identify areas of interest and, if appropriate, the intended biopsy site and safety range (with regards to depth as well as blood vessels and viscera in the vicinity).

4. Use the freehand technique to perform TTFNA of various pathologies. Make sure the patient does not alter position during the procedure, and use adequate local analgesia (to minimize pain and avoid sudden movements). Furthermore, avoid puncture of intercostal arteries (inferior to ribs), the internal thoracic/mammarian artery (1–2 cm lateral to the sternum), and subclavian and major intrathoracic vessels when attempting a biopsy.

5. Once a specimen is obtained by means of TTFNA, material should be expelled onto slides within seconds. The quality of smear preparation is as important as the biopsy technique.

6. Utilize ROSE to provisionally confirm the presence of diagnostic material.

7. Where epithelial carcinoma or an infectious process is not suspected or identified on ROSE, perform a CNB, provided a safety range can be guaranteed.

8. Always identify the diaphragm and subdiaphragmatic viscera prior to performing lower transthoracic biopsies, as these structures may be displaced cephalad, giving a false impression of a solid mass or consolidated lung.

9. Use the ultrasound to screen for post-procedural pneumothoraces.

CHAPTER 10

## REFERENCES

1. Koh D, Burke S, Davis N, et al. Transthoracic US of the chest: clinical uses and applications. *Radiographics* 2002; 22(1):e1.

2. Koegelenberg CFN, Bolliger CT, Diacon AH. Pleural ultrasound. In Light RW, Lee YC (eds.), *Textbook of pleural disease*, 2nd ed. London, Hodder & Stoughton, 2008: 275–83.

3. Koegelenberg CFN, Diacon AH, Bolliger CT. Transthoracic ultrasound of the chest wall, pleura, and the peripheral lung. In Bollger, CT, Herth FJF, Mayo PH, Miyazama T, Beamis JF (eds.), *Progress in respiratory research. Clinical chest ultrasound*, vol. 37. Basel, Karger, 2009: 22–33.

4. Hoosen MM, Barnes D, Khan AN, et al. The importance of ultrasound in staging and gaining a pathological diagnosis in patients with lung cancer—a two year single centre experience. *Thorax* 2011; 66:414–17.

5. Diacon AH, Schuurmans MM, Theron J, et al. Safety and yield of ultrasound assisted transthoracic biopsy performed by pulmonologists. *Respiration* 2004; 71:519–22.

6. Diacon AH, Theron J, Schubert P, et al. Ultrasound-assisted transthoracic biopsy: fine-needle aspiration or cutting-needle biopsy? *Eur Respir J* 2007; 29:357–62.

7. Koegelenberg CFN, Bolliger CT, Irusen EM, et al. The diagnostic yield and safety of ultrasound-assisted transthoracic fine needle aspiration of drowned lung. *Respiration* 2011; 81:26–31.

8. Lichtenstein D, Mézière G. A lung ultrasound sign allowing bedside distinction between pulmonary edema and COPD: the comet-tail artifact. *Intensive Care Med* 1998; 24:1331–34.

9. Lichtenstein D, Mézière G, Biderman P, Gepner A, Barré O. The comet-tail artifact: an ultrasound sign of alveolar–interstitial syndrome. *Am J Respir Crit Care Med* 1997; 156:1640–46.

10. Koegelenberg CF, Bolliger CT, Irusen EM, et al. The diagnostic yield and safety of ultrasound-assisted biopsy of mediastinal masses. *Respiration* 2011; 81:134–41.

11. Saito T, Kobayashi H, Sugama Y, et al. Ultrasonically guided needle biopsy in the diagnosis of mediastinal masses. *Am Rev Respir Dis* 1988; 138:679–684.

12. Yang PC, Chang DB, Yu CJ, et al. Ultrasound-guided core biopsy of thoracic tumors. *Am Rev Respir Dis* 1992; 146:763–767.

CHAPTER 10

### MCQ 1

**Q** A patient presents with progressive dyspnea, with the high-frequency ultrasound image shown right. Which of the following statements are true (multiple answers possible)?

**a.** The patient has a pneumothorax.

**b.** There is evidence of pulmonary edema.

**c.** There are prominent A lines.

**d.** There are prominent B lines.

**e.** A small pleural effusion is present.

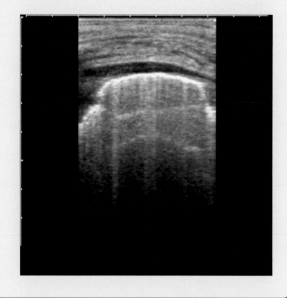

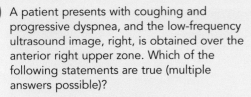

## MCQ 2

**Q** A patient presents with coughing and progressive dyspnea, and the low-frequency ultrasound image, right, is obtained over the anterior right upper zone. Which of the following statements are true (multiple answers possible)?

**a.** There are prominent B lines.

**b.** The patient has a pneumothorax.

**c.** There is evidence of pulmonary consolidation.

**d.** There is evidence of pulmonary edema.

**e.** Bronchograms can be observed.

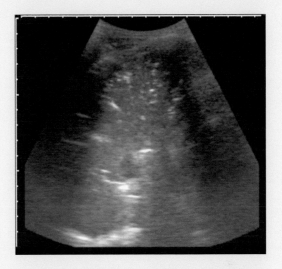

## MCQ 3

**Q** A patient presents with a peripheral pulmonary mass with no associated mediastinal lymphadenopathy or distant metastases. The ultrasound image is shown right. The tumor did not shift position with respiration. Which of the following statements are true (multiple answers possible)?

**a.** The tumor invades only the visceral pleura.

**b.** The tumor invades the parietal pleura and chest wall.

**c.** An ultrasound-assisted transthoracic fine-needle aspiration has a high diagnostic yield for lung cancer in this setting.

**d.** The acoustic window is too narrow to demonstrate the whole circumference of the lesion.

**e.** The acoustic window does not allow for the full depth of the lesion to be measured.

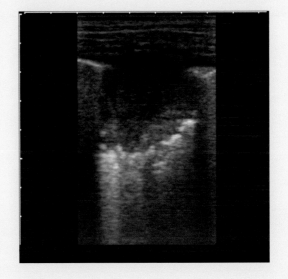

CHAPTER 10

## MCQ 4

 **Q** A patient presents with an anterior mediastinal mass and is subsequently referred for an ultrasound-assisted biopsy. Low-frequency ultrasound (right parasternal view) confirms the mass. Which of the following statements are true (multiple answers possible)?

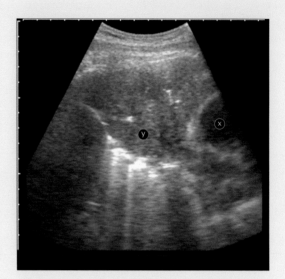

a. X is a great vessel.

b. Y represents a solid tumor mass.

c. An ultrasound-assisted transthoracic fine-needle aspiration has a high diagnostic yield for lung cancer in this setting.

d. An ultrasound-assisted transthoracic fine-needle aspiration has a greater than 90% diagnostic yield for lymphomas in this setting.

e. A cutting needle biopsy following a non-diagnostic TTFNA would be contraindicated in this particular case, given the vicinity of the large vessels.

## ANSWERS

 **A** **1.** b, d, e

See Chapter 10 for explanation

 **A** **2.** c,e

 **A** **3.** b, c, d

 **A** **4.** a, b, c

# Ultrasound Training and Accreditation

Amelia O. Clive and Nick A. Maskell

## INTRODUCTION

The use of thoracic ultrasound by non-radiology-trained clinicians is increasing ac ross the world, both in the diagnostic workup for pleural pathologies and for guiding invasive pleural procedures. In order for ultrasound to be performed safely and accurately, robust training and accreditation need to be available in order to maintain standards and ensure patient safety.

There is evidence that the use of ultrasound in guiding pleural procedures may help to minimize procedure-related complications[1–3] (see Chapter 1). With adequate training, respiratory physician-delivered thoracic ultrasound has been shown to be accurate and safe for the identification of pleural effusion and in choosing a site for intervention.[4] This, along with concerns about drain misplacement using a "blind" approach,[5] has led to current best practice guidelines advocating the use of thoracic ultrasound to guide pleural interventions involving fluid.[6] In addition, the decreasing cost of portable ultrasound machines has led to better availability of this technology, and hence more clinicians are eager to acquire this skill. Audit data would suggest that the majority of UK respiratory departments have access to at least one ultrasound machine.[7] However, simply having access to a machine is not sufficient, and adequate staff training is imperative to ensure the equipment is used correctly.

Clinicians from a variety of different fields may benefit from skills in thoracic ultrasound, and recommendations about training are included in guidelines for critical care physicians,[8] surgeons,[9] emergency medicine clinicians,[10] and respiratory physicians.[11,12]

## TEACHING METHODS

Ultrasound is operator dependent and requires both psychomotor and cognitive skills in order to obtain high-quality images and interpret them. Adequate training and hands-on experience are therefore required in order for operators to be sufficiently skilled in all of these areas.

The traditional "see one, do one, teach one" approach to teaching is increasingly being replaced by a multi-modality method, to include theory sessions, simulation, direct observation, and observed practice.[13] Many of the established introductory courses in thoracic ultrasound include all of these methods.[14–16] One study in the United States, which evaluated a simulation-based ultrasound training module for interns, found it improved trainees' confidence in identifying specific structures using ultrasound, and hence it is felt to be useful preparation for supervised clinical practice.[17]

A variety of simulation mannequins have been developed for ultrasound training to replicate normal anatomy as well as a variety of thoracic pathologies, including atelectatic lung and pleural effusions. They can help improve confidence in the early stages of ultrasound training and can also be used as an introduction to ultrasound-guided pleural procedures (Figures 11.1a and b). Self-made thoracic phantoms can also be created to simulate the appearance of normal lung and pleural pathology, which can be helpful for teaching diagnostic and procedural ultrasound.

It is well known that the rate at which people learn practical procedures varies, and hence training schedules may need to be individually tailored. All the

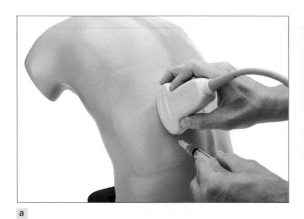

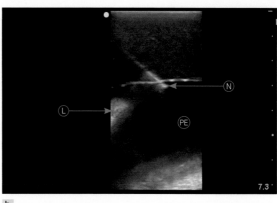

a

b

**Figure 11.1** (a) Blue Phantom thoracentesis ultrasound simulation model. Allows teaching of ultrasound-guided pleural effusion assessment and real-time aspiration. (b) Associated ultrasound image demonstrating visualization of the pleural effusion (PE) and aspiration needle (N). L = lung. (Courtesy of Blue Phantom, Redmond, Washington, www.bluephantom.com)

training syllabuses include a list of specific competencies that must be obtained prior to certification being granted,[14,18–20] in addition to a minimum period of observed practice.

Given the potentially complex anatomy and range of pathologies that can be identified using thoracic ultrasound, it is important that trainees have sufficient experience of a variety of normal and pathological cases during their training. Regardless of the number of scans performed, it is important that the person certifying a trainee is convinced that he or she has sufficient training and practical experience of ultrasound to be competent and safe to perform the technique unsupervised.

It is also recognized that some clinicians require more in-depth skills and experience than others, for example, in order to train other colleagues in the technique, perform directly guided invasive procedures, and undertake research in ultrasound. This has led to the development of different levels of competence in many of the training recommendations[18,19] (Table 11.1).

However, despite the increasing use of thoracic ultrasound and the benefits it can confer with regard to patient safety, it is still felt that there are some barriers to training. One American study used an online tool to survey critical care and pulmonary program directors and found 74% of programs offered lung and pleural ultrasound training.[21] Impediments to training that were identified included high rate of fellow turnover, lack of access to an ultrasound machine, and financial constraints.[21]

**Table 11.1 British and European competency levels for thoracic ultrasound[18,19]**

**Level 1**
- To perform common examinations safely and accurately
- To recognize and differentiate normal anatomy and pathology
- To diagnose common abnormalities
- To recognize when a referral for a second opinion is indicated
- To understand the relationship between ultrasound imaging and other diagnostic imaging techniques (UK only)

**Level 2**
- To accept and manage referrals from Level 1 practitioners
- To recognize and diagnose almost all conditions within the relevant organ system
- To perform common noncomplex ultrasound-guided invasive procedures
- To teach ultrasound to trainees and Level 1 practitioners
- To conduct some research in ultrasound)

**Level 3**—advanced level of practice, including some or all of:
- To accept tertiary referrals from Level 1 and 2 practitioners
- To perform specialized ultrasound examinations
- To perform advanced ultrasound-guided invasive procedures
- To conduct substantial research in ultrasound
- To teach ultrasound at all levels
- To be aware of and pursue developments in ultrasound

# THE FUTURE OF ULTRASOUND TRAINING

In the first instance, the expansion of training opportunities and availability of ultrasound machines are important to ensure basic competence is obtained by more physicians undertaking pleural interventions. As pressure increases for doctors to prove competence at procedures and demonstrate ongoing proficiency after initial training, the guidelines for thoracic ultrasound training may become more rigorous.

As use of ultrasound by non-radiology-trained clinicians expands for a variety of clinical indications (including echocardiography, vascular and abdominal imaging) and technology becomes more portable (for example, the advent of handheld ultrasound devices), there may be a role for the acquisition of basic ultrasound skills to begin in medical schools. By incorporating it into the undergraduate curriculum, this would allow newly qualified doctors to have basic competence that could be subsequently developed during specialist training.

# SPECIFIC TRAINING REQUIREMENTS AROUND THE WORLD

Minimum training requirements for thoracic ultrasound have been developed by a number of organizations around the world to formalize the training process and ensure clinicians using this technology are competent.

The specific training requirements and competencies for the various schemes and levels differ between organizations (see Table 11.2, next page), but there are a number of common themes, which are included in all of the programs.[18–20,22] These include:

- Knowledge regarding the physics and technology. of ultrasound and ultrasound techniques.
- Normal sectional and ultrasonic anatomy.
- Thoracic pathology in relation to ultrasound.

The American College of Chest Physicians (ACCP) incorporates thoracic ultrasound training into a more general critical care ultrasound program, which also includes vascular and abdominal ultrasound and echocardiography.[16] It defines specific technical and cognitive competencies required in order to be certified,[20] and trainees must submit an online portfolio of ultrasound images and be successful in a written examination.[16] The Accreditation Council for Graduate Medical Education (ACGME) in the United States has specified ultrasound-guided thoracentesis as a required competency in its 2012 curriculum for respiratory and critical care trainees.[12]

The British, Australasian, and European requirements for basic accreditation involve attendance at a training course, supervised practice, and the acquisition of specific competencies. The European and British systems subdivide the accreditation process into three levels of training and expertise[18,23] (see Table 11.1). Level 2 accreditation requires at least 1 year's practical experience of thoracic ultrasound (after obtaining level 1). In the UK, clinicians must also have performed a further 100 thoracic ultrasounds during this time, but in Europe a further 300 examinations are required in order to be awarded level 2. Level 3 training is really the remit of experts in the area, including practitioners who spend the majority of their time undertaking ultrasound or specialist thoracic radiologists.

# CONTINUOUS PROFESSIONAL DEVELOPMENT

Once a level of competency has been attained, it is important that skills are maintained for continuous professional development (CPD). This will involve performing regular examinations (and recording them in a logbook), auditing practice, and keeping up to date with the published literature.[14,18,23]

Clinicians should have ongoing access to mentors with level 2 or 3 accreditation, after they have been awarded initial certification. Some national guidelines have also advocated this approach.[18] Mentors can help by reviewing saved ultrasound images, assist in challenging cases, and support the development of more advanced skills, such as the use of advanced ultrasound techniques (e.g., Doppler) and real-time guided pleural procedures.

Table 11.2 Training requirements and minimum number of ultrasound examinations to be observed and performed to achieve level 1 ultrasound training (or equivalent) for different accreditation schemes

| Organization | Attendance at training course required? | Number of ultrasounds to be observed | Total minimum number of supervised ultrasounds performed | Minimum number of supervised ultrasounds showing pathology performed | Minimum number of pleural procedures using ultrasound guidance | End-of-training certification | Minimum number of ultrasounds per year to maintain certification at level 1 |
|---|---|---|---|---|---|---|---|
| Australasian Society for Ultrasound in Medicine[22] | Yes (course in applied physics and instrumentation and thoracic ultrasound course of at least 3 hours) | Not specified | 20 (at least 3 directly observed; the remaining images to be reviewed by an experienced sonographer) | 5 | 5 (using indirect US guidance) | Awarded by the ASUM Council upon submission of documentation that all requirements have been met | Not specified |
| The Royal College of Radiologists, UK (level 1)[18] | Yes (duration of course not specified) | Not specified | At least 1 session per week over a period of at least 3 months, with ~5 scans per session performed by trainee under supervision | Examinations should encompass the full range of specific pathological conditions | Not specified | Local sign-off by level 2 practitioner (or higher) once competencies and logbook completed | 20 |
| European Federation of Societies for Ultrasound in Medicine and Biology (level 1)[19] | Yes (minimum 15 hours) | 25 | 200 (at least 100 examinations on normal patients) | 50 effusions | 25 | Local sign-off by trainer once competencies and logbook completed | 100 |
| ACCP Certificate of Completion Critical Care Ultrasonography Program[16] | Yes (attendance at a variety of courses encompassing fundamentals of ultrasound and specific anatomical areas) | Not specified | 20 (including 5 normal examinations) | 10 effusions 5 consolidations | Not specified | Awarded by ACCP if meets requirements and successful in end-of-training exam (includes other types of critical care US) | Not specified |

ASUM = Australasian Society of Ultrasound in Medicine, ACCP = American College of Chest Physicians, US = ultrasound.

# CONCLUSION

Thoracic ultrasound is an expanding area. It can provide useful clinical information at the bedside and has the potential to improve the safety of thoracic procedures. In order to maintain standards and ensure patient safety, it is important that a training infrastructure is established to support its use by non-radiology-trained clinicians. Emphasis must be placed on competence at both image acquisition and interpretation when awarding certification. It is also important that clinicians have ongoing access to advice and assistance from experienced radiology colleagues throughout their training and after accreditation has been granted.

**TIPS FOR CLINICAL PRACTICE**

- Ensure you have a local radiology mentor to help you with difficult cases.
- Keep a logbook of all the ultrasounds you perform as evidence of CPD.
- Save images for review with your mentor at a later date.
- Consider finding a buddy during your ultrasound training to work with and compare images and interpretations.
- Audit your practice.
- Keep up to date with current practice and literature on thoracic ultrasound.

# REFERENCES

1. Gordon CE, Feller-Kopman D, Balk EM, Smetana GW. Pneumothorax following thoracentesis: a systematic review and meta-analysis. *Archives of Internal Medicine* 2010; 170(4):332–39.

2. Duncan DR, Morgenthaler TI, Ryu JH, Daniels CE. Reducing iatrogenic risk in thoracentesis: establishing best practice via experiential training in a zero-risk environment. *Chest* 2009; 135(5):1315–20.

3. Diacon AH, Brutsche MH, Soler M. Accuracy of pleural puncture sites: a prospective comparison of clinical examination with ultrasound. *Chest* 2003; 123(2):436–41.

4. Rahman NM, Singanayagam A, Davies HE, Wrightson JM, Mishra EK, Lee YC, et al. Diagnostic accuracy, safety and utilisation of respiratory physician-delivered thoracic ultrasound. *Thorax* 2010; 65(5):449–53.

5. National Patient Safety Agency. Risks of chest drain insertion. NPSA/2008/RRR003. 2008. Available from www.npsa.nhs.uk/patientsafety/alerts-and-directives (accessed May 15, 2008).

6. Havelock T, Teoh R, Laws D, Gleeson F. Pleural procedures and thoracic ultrasound: British Thoracic Society Pleural Disease guideline 2010. *Thorax* 2010; 65(Suppl 2):ii61–76.

7. Hooper C, Maskell N. British Thoracic Society national pleural procedures audit 2010. *Thorax* 2011;66(7):636–37.

8. American Board of Internal Medicine. Critical care medicine policies. 2012. Available from www.abim.org/certification/policies/imss/ccm.aspx (accessed February 15, 2012).

9. American College of Surgeons. Ultrasound examinations by surgeons. 1998. Available from www.facs.org/fellows_info/statements/st-31.html (accessed January 11, 2012).

10. American College of Emergency Physicians. Use of ultrasound imaging by emergency physicians. *Annals of Emergency Medicine* 2001; 38(4):469–70.

11. Joint Royal Colleges of Physicians Training Board. Specialty training curriculum for respiratory medicine. 2010. Available from www.jrcptb.org.uk/specialties/ST3-SpR/Documents/2010%20Respiratory%20Medicine%20Curriculum.pdf (accessed February 15, 2012).

12. Accreditation Council for Graduate Medical Education. ACGME program requirements for graduate medical education in pulmonary disease (internal medicine). 2012. Available from www.acgme.org/acWebsite/downloads/RRC_progReq/149_pulmonary_disease_int_Med_07012012.pdf.

13. Lenchus JD, Birnbach DJ. Rethinking invasive procedural training. Academic medicine. *Journal of the Association of American Medical Colleges* 2010; 85(4):570.

14. Australasian Society for Ultrasound in Medicine. Certificate in clinician performed ultrasound (CCPU). Available from http://www.asum.com.au/newsite/Education.php?p=CCPU.

15. British Thoracic Society. BTS thoracic ultrasound short course. 2012. Available from www.brit-thoracic.org.uk/bts-learning-hub/short-courses/thoracic-ultrasound-bristol.aspx (accessed February 14, 2012).

16. ACCP. Certificate of completion critical care ultrasonography program. 2011. Available from www.chestnet.org/accp/accp-certificate-completion-critical-care-ultrasonography-program (accessed December 5, 2011).

17. Keddis MT, Cullen MW, Reed DA, Halvorsen AJ, McDonald FS, Takahashi PY, et al. Effectiveness of an ultrasound training module for internal medicine residents. *BMC Medical Education* 2011; 11:75.

18. Board of the Faculty of Clinical Radiology. Ultrasound training recommendations for medical and sugical specialties. 2004. Available from http://www.rcr.ac.uk/docs/radiology/pdf/ultrasound.pdf.

19. European Federation of Societies for Ultrasound in Medicine and Biology. Minimum training requirements for the practice of medical ultrasound in Europe. Appendix 11: Thoracic ultrasound. 2008. Available from www.efsumb.org/guidelines/2009-04-14apx11.pdf (accessed February 10, 2012).

20. Mayo PH, Beaulieu Y, Doelken P, Feller-Kopman D, Harrod C, Kaplan A, et al. American College of Chest Physicians/La Société de Réanimation de Langue Française statement on competence in critical care ultrasonography. *Chest* 2009; 135(4):1050–60.

21. Eisen LA, Leung S, Gallagher AE, Kvetan V. Barriers to ultrasound training in critical care medicine fellowships: a survey of program directors. *Critical Care Medicine* 2010; 38(10):1978–83.

22. Australasian Society for Ultrasound in Medicine. Certificate in clinician performed ultrasound (CCPU) short syllabus. Unit: pleural effusion. 2011. Available from www.asum.com.au/newsite/files/Documents/Education/CCPU/CCPU%20Syllabus/Pleural%20effusion_2011.pdf (accessed February 15, 2012).

23. European Federation of Societies for Ultrasound in Medicine and Biology. Minimum training recommendations for the practice of medical ultrasound. 2007. Available from www.efsumb.org/uploads/mintraining-Feb2006.pdf (accessed February 10, 2012).

# Choosing a Thoracic Ultrasound Machine

Rahul Bhatnagar, Anthony Edey, and Nick Maskell

## INTRODUCTION

Selecting and purchasing an ultrasound machine for a respiratory department is a decision that should be undertaken with as much preparation as possible. There can be a wealth of technical information to absorb, and an imposing choice of manufacturers and suppliers. This section aims to enable the reader to approach purchasing decisions in a relevant, systematic fashion. Although international variation in manufacturer and model availability means much of the following information is generic, the core messages remain the same regardless of location. These begin with ensuring that adequate time is spent researching and choosing equipment, and that at the heart of any decision there is a necessary compromise between budget, machine versatility, and the technology available.

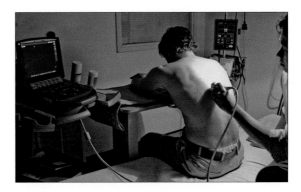

**Figure 12.1** An example of a bedside thoracic ultrasound examination with adequate space for machine and operator.

12

## TECHNICAL FACTORS

### Proposed use and setting

The basic principles of ultrasound examination and diagnostics remain the same regardless of the clinical setting. However, as the use of this modality has spread across medicine and its subspecialities, manufacturers have sought to adapt their technology to progressively smaller areas. Respiratory medicine has the potential to overlap many of these niches, and so it is important to be clear about the scope of intended use. The most basic of machines with a simple linear probe may be used for peripheral and central line insertion (in conjunction with Doppler function), but will be insufficient for anything other than detailed examination of the pleura in a slim patient, and will have a very limited field of view. A low-frequency curvilinear probe allows a broader overview of the thorax, including the pleura, effusions, and nonaerated segments of lung, as well as being capable of abdominal and pelvic examination. Separate, dedicated probes are required for formal cardiac examination, though a "small footprint" phased-array transducer can be an excellent probe to image the pleura, lung, heart, and abdominal structures.

The layout, design, and organization of a hospital or clinic will also have a significant practical impact on the type of machine that should be considered. A dedicated outpatient environment or thoracic procedure room may facilitate the purchase of a stationary yet more complex machine. Conversely, and perhaps more typically, imaging and procedures take place in a variety of settings and require a more portable device (Figure 12.1).

## Size

Scanner size varies considerably and, broadly speaking, is proportional to processing power and thus cost. Far more portable, sometimes handheld, equipment has become available in recent years. Small-scale scanners (Figure 12.2) are ideal for point-of-care use (including rapid response teams) and guided interventions, but are often able to work with only one type of probe and have small, lower-resolution screens. Many have limited functionality, and those that are more versatile may be less user-friendly because of the lack of space for a keyboard, additional buttons, or connectors. At the other extreme are ultrasound machines whose large size make movement between locations impractical and which often need to be fixed to one site; these are typically the domain of radiology departments (Figure 12.3). Large machines will often have complete flexibility in function and excellent image processing, but require the patient to attend the location of the machine if it is to be used to its full potential. Inevitably, high-end, large scanners are considerably more expensive than smaller, less sophisticated alternatives.

In practice, a compromise between size, functionality, and image quality is required, and this may be achieved by a mid-size scanner. Similar in appearance to a large laptop computer, these machines are often able to provide some complex functions and the ability to swap between a limited selection of probes. These devices have been found, in the authors' experience, to be the most practical for general respiratory use (Figures 12.4 and 12.5). While not designed to be used in a handheld fashion, they are extremely portable and can be readily moved to the patient's bedside. Practical downsides of portability are the vulnerability of expensive equipment to theft, as well as making them prone to accidental damage during transportation. Thus, designating a safe storage space is an important consideration for equipment protection in the long term.

The ideal solution to transportation and positioning during scanning is that devices should be bought with an appropriate stand. Stands need to be adjustable to ensure the physician is comfortable while both scanning and performing interventions to prevent back injuries (Figure 12.6).

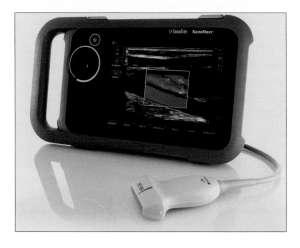

**Figure 12.2** A small, high-end handheld ultrasound machine shown with a linear probe. (Product picture supplied by SonoSite, Inc., Bothell, Washington.)

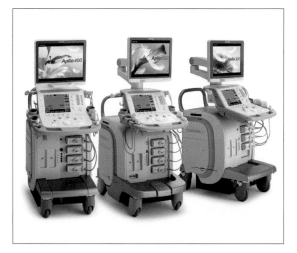

**Figure 12.3** A range of large, high-end ultrasound machines. (Product picture supplied by Toshiba Medical Systems.)

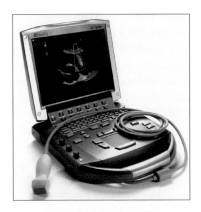

**Figure 12.4** (left) A mid-sized, mid-range portable ultrasound machine, shown with a phased transducer. (Product picture supplied by SonoSite, Inc., Bothell, Washington.)

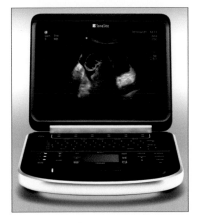

**Figure 12.5** (left) A mid-sized, high-end portable ultrasound machine. (Product picture supplied by SonoSite, Inc., Bothell, Washington.)

**Figure 12.6** (right) An ultrasound machine attached to a dedicated stand. Shown with a phased transducer and printer. (Product picture supplied by SonoSite, Inc., Bothell, Washington.)

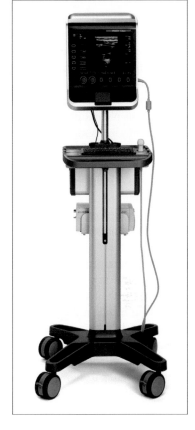

## Battery life and power source

It is unusual for a patient to undergo a pleural procedure without a nearby power source, but sometimes there may be need to use an ultrasound machine from battery alone. It is important to quantify the potential usage time in this setting, as well as the standby time without being connected to main power. For more portable machines, check if a power brick is required (this may limit their versatility), and if it is possible to buy additional batteries. One should also ensure a manufacturer states how long it expects a battery to last with repeated use and charging, and, if purchasing from overseas, whether the machine will run using the voltage and frequency of the local power supply. Additionally, one should know the "boot-up time" of the unit being considered, as this can vary from a few seconds to close to a minute.

## Image storage or printing

Being able to quickly and easily store or print images taken on a machine is a useful feature. Many departments will require this facility for audit trails, as well as for training, educational, and billing purposes. The ideal solution is that images can be stored directly on a picture archiving and communication system (PACS) as part of the patient's formal imaging record. In reality, this level of connectivity can be problematic and simpler alternatives may be required. Thus, it is important to know if the device can store images, and whether these are in a commonly used format such as JPEG. In addition, it is important to confirm that, once stored, images can be easily extracted from the memory using ubiquitous connectors such as universal serial bus (USB).

## Screen and image processing

The widespread availability of cheap, flat monitors and screens has in no small part aided the proliferation of portable ultrasound. However, small screens may be difficult to see, particularly in bright clinical areas, and may be limited by low spatial resolution, preventing adequate depiction of subtle abnormalities, such as pleural nodularity. Large-screen devices are inherently less portable, and although they do allow for greater screen quality, one should remember that a larger screen is not a guarantee of image fidelity. In practice, image quality is the result of many factors, including transducer quality, system processing power, and the inherent resolution of the monitor. Of these factors, the processing power of a system is the principal determinant of cost, and larger housing usually allows for more processing power at a lower cost, in much the same way as an equivalent laptop computer will cost more than its desktop counterpart. Figure 12.7 attempts to highlight the potential difference between high-end and mid-range machines. The authors would recommend that devices are tested, or at least viewed in action, before purchase, and in fact, many manufacturers will be willing to allow trial periods of use before a full purchase is made.

## Probe compatibility and range

The more probes available for a particular machine, the more versatile the machine may be. For many mid- and high-end machines, it is usually possible to purchase additional transducers at a later date. This allows for future expansion of functionality, depending on clinical need, and may be more attractive than purchasing all components initially. Much of the technology that allows an ultrasound to operate is housed in the transducer, and so one should expect to pay a reasonable premium for each one. Larger machines often allow multiple probes to be connected simultaneously (Figure 12.8), which reduces the chance of damage and is more convenient if switching between examination types in one location.

**Figure 12.7** Image processing comparison. The same images from the same patient have been taken on two separate machines. The left-hand images are from a typical mid-range laptop-sized machine; the right-hand images are from a high-end, radiology department-based machine. The higher spatial resolution on the right-hand images allows for greater image clarity and more detailed examination.

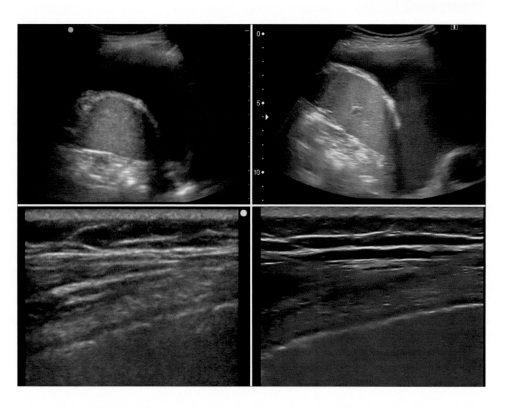

## Frequency range and modes

The typical range of frequencies needed for diagnostic ultrasound examination is between 2 and 18 megahertz (MHz). At the higher end of this range, ultrasound wave penetration is poor, but the spatial resolution, and thus ability to discern fine detail, is greatly improved. Higher-frequency probes tend to have a linear design and are often useful for guiding percutaneous line insertion, or for resolving visceral and parietal pleural motion. General thoracic examination requires a lower-frequency range of 3.5–5 MHz, as this allows deep structures and pleural effusions to be assessed in a wide field of view. Transducers in this range are usually curvilinear (convex) in shape.

Ultrasound can generate a variety of different data according to the mode of use. The most commonly used mode is B mode (brightness mode), which is standard on most machines and for the majority of situations will suffice, although Doppler analysis, both color and spectral, can also be useful in thoracic ultrasound. Preempting the range of applications a machine will be used for, as described earlier, will allow an appropriate purchase without the wasted expense of underutilized functionality.

## The "ideal" respiratory ultrasound

Table 12.1 suggests characteristics that, in the authors' experience, should be considered mandatory when choosing an ultrasound device. Potentially desirable characteristics are also included, although these will vary between centers according to use.

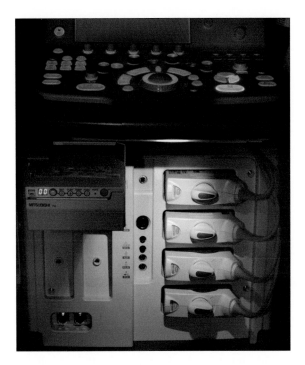

**Figure 12.8** Multiple probes are shown connected to a high-end machine (illuminated on the bottom right of the image), allowing greater versatility. (Image supplied by Toshiba Medical Systems.)

CHAPTER 12

**Table 12.1 Characteristics to consider when choosing a thoracic ultrasound machine**

| Mandatory characteristics | Desirable characteristics |
| --- | --- |
| Low-frequency curvilinear probe | Additional linear probe, or ability to add probes at a later date |
| Basic functionality, such as gain adjustment and depth measurement | Doppler function |
| Ability to operate over both high and low frequencies | Ability to run off batteries |
| Image storage and extraction capability | Ability to upload images to PACS |
| Screen with size and spatial resolution to allow viewing from at least 2–3 ft (60–90 cm) away | High spatial resolution flat screen of largest practical size |
| Mobility adequate to allow bedside examination | QWERTY keyboard |
| | Ability to record video |

# COST FACTORS

## Unit and probe costs

Although the majority of the costs of an ultrasound machine will likely be made up of the machine itself, one must remember there are many extra purchasing decisions that must be factored in. An important question to ask early on is: How many machines are needed? Many smaller departments will function adequately with a single scanner, but this becomes limiting if there is the need for multiple simultaneous exams, or if the device develops a fault. Although the initial outlay will be higher, manufacturers or suppliers may be willing to offer discounts for bulk purchases, which improves value for money.

As mentioned earlier, transducer probes can be expensive items in themselves. It is important to ensure that the appropriate probes are included in any package under consideration, and to be clear on the costs of purchasing additional probes in the future. Similarly, understanding the intended use of any machine should help to avoid purchasing probes that will rarely see use. One should also note that the same unit can be sold with several software packages, and it is important to purchase the required ones, but also be able to upgrade as your skill and sonographic examinations become more sophisticated.

Table 12.2 illustrates typical cost ranges for components and machines of varying types. Costs are based on UK 2012 estimates and may vary internationally.

## Ways to lower purchasing costs

Although purchasing the latest machine may seem desirable, the limited nature of respiratory ultrasound examination when compared to, for example, obstetrics means that many of the latest machines will house features that will never be used. Many suppliers will offer units that are 1 or 2 years old at significantly reduced rates, with no particular detriment to their use in thoracic examination. Local departments with a higher turnover of machines, such as cardiology or radiology, may also be able to offer used devices at lower rates. If considering a preowned machine, it is vital to ensure that all appropriate service checks have been made and that there have been no serious faults.

Options to spread the costs of ultrasound machines may also be available. Although lower monthly costs may be attractive, finance agreements will typically include interest, which may make the overall fee payable greater than if the total cost was paid up front. Although long-term finance agreements may limit the scope for later expansion or addition of functionality, some may offer the option of regular upgrades to the latest equipment.

**Table 12.2 Breakdown of estimated costs of thoracic ultrasound equipment**

| Item | Cost range (US$) |
| --- | --- |
| Smaller handheld ultrasound machine | 7000–10,000 |
| High-end handheld ultrasound machine | 10,000–20,000 |
| Standard, mid-size (laptop) ultrasound machine | 30,000–50,000 |
| High-end, mid-size (laptop) ultrasound machine | 50,000–100,000 |
| Standard, large ultrasound machine | 30,000–70,000 |
| High-end, large ultrasound machine | 75,000–150,000 |
| Transducer probe | 5000–10,000 |
| Annual service contract | ~10 of purchase price |
| Photo printer | ~1000 |
| Portable stand | 200–500 |

CHAPTER 12

**TIPS FOR CLINICAL PRACTICE**

- Purchasing an ultrasound machine will often be a compromise between functionality and cost.
- Establish the intended setting for use and storage, as well as how the machine will be used clinically, as this will help to determine machine size and complexity.
- Look to use a new machine for a trial period before committing to a significant purchase, or perhaps consider a used machine at a lower cost.
- Beware of hidden costs over and above the initial outlay—service plans, parts, training, and consumables should all be considered.

## Service plan and technical support

Thoracic ultrasound machines will typically undergo regular use, be moved frequently, and be used by a variety of personnel. It is therefore vital to ensure a suitable service plan is in place to cover parts and unit failure. When considering a service plan, check whether it includes regular inspections, whether ancillary components such as probes and batteries are covered, and whether repair due to accidental damage is included. The provision of technical support should also be taken into account during purchase. If a device should experience a problem, will the supplier or manufacturer attempt to repair it on site, or will they arrange for the machine to be taken away? Some may require the user to arrange transport, thus incurring extra costs. Check whether an alternative machine can be supplied during repair times, and whether there is a geographical limit to the service arrangements being offered. The latter point is especially important if machines are to be used in less well-connected hospitals. If manufacturer service plans are not suitable or competitive, or they are not available on used machines, third-party service and warranty agreements are often available.

## Training costs

Although perhaps not an immediate thought when purchasing an ultrasound device, the costs of training users should always be factored in to overall projections. Manufacturers will often offer a simple educational session to allow users to become oriented with a device, but more detailed courses may be needed to ensure machines are used to their full potential. Purchasers should also consider the costs of mandatory training and accreditation, which will often be necessary before examinations can be done in a clinical setting.

## Other considerations

There are numerous minor and ongoing costs that may exist following purchase of an ultrasound machine. Departments should budget for consumables such as ultrasound transmission gel, extra batteries, and photo or printer paper if applicable. Resale value may be an issue if there are plans for regular upgrades, and shipping and installation costs should also be made clear at the outset.

When deciding upon a machine, it may also be worth enlisting the help of those who are already familiar with the nuances of ultrasound operation. The most useful opinions are likely to be those of ultrasonographers, ideally those with specialist thoracic interest. Asking such colleagues to give advice or to trial machines alongside respiratory physicians may help to reveal subtleties that would otherwise only become apparent with prolonged use.

## CONCLUSION

The decision to purchase an ultrasound machine for thoracic use can be complicated, but by following basic principles and exploring the market, purchasers can ensure that the appropriate device is obtained within budget and without hidden costs, ensuring long-term benefit to departments, operators, and ultimately, patients.

CHAPTER 12

# Index

Note: Page references in *italic* refer to E-book video or ultrasound clips.

## C